Metaphors of Memory

Dr Natwar Sharma is an associate professor in paediatrics and paediatric critical care. He is currently on a sabbatical, in Kuwait.

Dr Sharma is a member of the Royal College of Paediatrics and Child Health (UK) and has served and trained at the Apollo Hospitals, Chennai. He has had an excellent academic career and was awarded the national gold medal for paediatrics in 2006, by the National Board of Examinations.

During his studies, Dr Sharma encountered certain anomalies for which mainstream medicine had no answer. This made him probe deeper into the cause and origin of diseases and opened his vision to alternative and holistic therapies of healing. He ended up discovering the science of regression therapy, which he combines with his practice of mainstream medicine. He hopes to bring about a paradigm shift in the field of health by bridging these conventional and non-conventional techniques of healing.

He is a certified member of the Earth Association for Regression Therapy and a certified teacher of transpersonal regression therapy. He has been presenting his research work at the World Congress for Regression Therapy since 2011. A trainer of the Heartfulness system of meditation, Dr Sharma is currently studying the effects of meditation on the body, mind, brain, heart and aura.

Metaphors of Memory

Healing Through Past and Current Life Regression

A Doctor's Perspective

DR NATWAR SHARMA

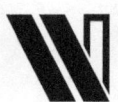

First published by Westland Publications Private Limited in 2021

Published by Westland Books, a division of Nasadiya Technologies Private Limited, in 2023

No. 269/2B, First Floor, 'Irai Arul', Vimalraj Street, Nethaji Nagar, Alapakkam Main Road, Maduravoyal, Chennai 600095

Westland and the Westland logo are the trademarks of Nasadiya Technologies Private Limited, or its affiliates..

Copyright © Dr Natwar Sharma, 2021.

ISBN: 9789357767552

10 9 8 7 6 5 4 3 2 1

The views and opinions expressed in this work are the author's own and the facts are as reported by him, and the publisher is in no way liable for the same.

All rights reserved

Typeset by Jojy Philip, New Delhi - 110015
Printed at Saurabh Printers Pvt. Ltd.

No part of this book may be reproduced, or stored in a retrieval system, or transmitted in any form or by any means, electronic, mechanical, photocopying, recording, or otherwise, without express written permission of the publisher.

Contents

Preface   vii

I. PREMISES

The Physical—and Beyond   3

The Scope of Regression Therapy   10
Vis-à-vis Mainstream Medicine

The Nature and Time of Healing   15

II. CASE STUDIES

A Sense of Insecurity   23
One Common Cause for Several Psychosomatic Conditions

Where Does the War End?   45
A Perspective on Chronic Conditions

We Are Not Only Our Genes   67
The Role of Epigenetics in Causing Health Disorders, Obesity, Diabetes and Hypertension

The Power of the Subconscious   81
Mental Conditioning Behind the Physical Condition

The Cord of Love 99
Regression in Children Through Surrogacy

In the Wake of Wisdom 111
Treating Multiple Disorders in an Individual Through Regression

III. ADDENDUM

Questions and Answers on Regression Therapy 159

IV. INSIGHT

The Science of Mind Over Matter 181

Acknowledgements 185

Preface

'Every human being has the right to ask the reason, why, and to have his question answered by himself, if he only takes the trouble.'

I came across these lines from the introductory chapter of Swami Vivekananda's book *Raja Yoga*, one afternoon in South India, in the summer of 2017. Around the same time, I wondered how to introduce my book, that had begun to take shape, to my readers. As I read the lines of this venerable modern mystic, I knew I had found the bridge to connect the intent behind the contents of my book and the way they may be perceived by the audience, who may or may not be a part of the medical fraternity to which I belong.

I believe the experiences in this book may be of great help to all those interested in supplementing their treatment regimens with holistic therapies that go beyond the physical realm. My medical fraternity may view the contents as evidence, providing them with the impetus to open up to regression therapy as a complementary non-conventional mode of treatment. And for the readers of this book, Vivekananda's words would motivate them and satisfy their curiosity enough to transport them to a different dimension—the spirit of inquiry, which is the essence of this book.

I am humbled that inspiration comes from none other than a Yogi who was, metaphorically speaking, a bridge between philosophy and practicality, a synthesis of science and spirituality, a passage between youthful enthusiasm and ancient wisdom, and a perfect blend of the Eastern way of feeling and the Western way of thinking. I could not have asked for a better opening, since the central theme of most of the cases shared in this book is that of healing through the bridge between metaphors from memories of the past and treatment of diseases in the present.

Starting my journey purely as a sceptic in the field of regression therapy, the more I became open to explore, the more I discovered. And the more I found and explored the radical and wonderful prospects that this non-conventional form of therapy could bring to the field of mainstream medicine, the more I sensed an urge to share its benefits with everybody. I hope that many minds open up to embrace this form of treatment—more as a complement to mainstream medicine than as a substitute for it.

As a child, my inquisitive nature had led me to discover that the mightiest trees are contained in the tiniest of seeds. In some mysterious fashion, this discovery gave me a small glimpse of the bigger picture of life, which, in turn, facilitated the acceptance and understanding of people and situations. Of course, over time I also realised that many of my 'whys' did not have answers in the world around me and that, in those cases, my quest had to take a different direction altogether. If my readers are apprehensive of a detour at this point, rest assured that I do not intend to make one in the least. This recollection of my childhood fascination is only to introduce the approach that I carry in my profession and is reflected in my clients' experiences, glimpses of which you will find surfacing time and again through the chapters of this book.

I don't know whether the habit influenced the dream or vice versa, but my nature of probing into things matured with time and I dreamed of becoming a detective when I grew up. While childhood dreams may mostly be a reflection of our fantasies that tend to melt away in the face of reality, old habits die hard. After graduating from medical school, I specialised in paediatrics and then trained as a paediatric intensivist. I went on to complete my MRCPCH from London, UK, after which I felt quite content as if there was little more to be done in life. As I started and got involved in my job as a practising paediatrician, I observed some striking aspects of mainstream medicine.

I realised that while the scope of mainstream medicine is vast, in several cases, it is almost irreplaceable. Imagine a situation where a person suffering from anaphylaxis is in immediate need of adrenaline and other fluids as first aid and is offered an alternative treatment by the physician instead. In this case, both the patient and the doctor are goners. *Nothing can replace intensive care and emergency medicine when the patient needs them.* At the same time, I also observed that mainstream medicine did have its limitations. It addressed the 'what' and 'how' of the manifesting issue in the patients by diagnosing the symptoms and pathogenesis of the disease. But it failed to address the 'why' part of the disease in many cases.

Over the course of my studies and practice, I noticed that the same disease could manifest in different ways and grades in different patients. Different patients may not respond to the same medication or treatment similarly in all cases. Sometimes, patients who seemed to have no hope of surviving made a miraculous recovery, while others who could have healed easily succumbed to the illness. Another intriguing fact was that not only did some patients exhibit greater resistance towards contracting diseases, but some of them were even able to communicate better with their bodies and facilitate their own recovery better than others.

To find the meaning behind these apparent anomalies, I started to broaden my perspective of therapeutics by looking at various alternative and complementary therapies. In the process, I stumbled upon the science of regression therapy. Initially, my judgement was clouded with doubt and disbelief. Being a person with a primarily scientific bent of mind, I needed evidence of the efficacy of any practice to embrace it wholeheartedly. Over time, prejudice gave way to conviction, with the emergence of first-hand evidence, and I gradually started discovering a new dimension to healing. What excited me the most is that I did not have to give up one for another, rather it was the combination of the conventional and the non-conventional that made all the difference.

My friends from the medical fraternity may wonder why we even need to address the 'why' of the disease. Instead of answering this question directly here, I urge them to read through the chapters and the cases presented with an open mind and discover the answer for themselves. It is not my intention in the least to dwell upon the limitations of mainstream medicine. Rather, I dare say that regression can actually enhance the scope of mainstream medicine in a very big way. If doctors can combine both the methods of healing—their own medical training along with this deep probing method—it can bring about a phenomenal and radical revolution in the field of health and medicine.

Even if you seek to explore the various dimensions of holistic healing and communicate better with your own physical body, the first step would be to understand the dynamics of body and mind, about disease and recovery. By being familiar with the nuances of regression, you become aware that healing through this therapy is neither mumbo-jumbo nor magic performed at the wave of a wand by the therapist. The premises and case studies presented in this book will help you to open up and understand the fact that regression—either to a past life or to a past time in the current life—works at a deeper level than the merely physical, and the client's cooperation and willing participation is equally important in integrating the effects of this form of treatment facilitated by the therapist.

This book intends to present all my work for readers at large to study with a spirit of scientific inquiry. In a way, it is also an invitation to the medical fraternity to be open and inspired to conduct deeper research and study this mode of therapy, to be convinced with the evidences that arise, and bring about a paradigm shift in mainstream medicine, collectively and consciously. The chapters of the book follow an evolutionary course, beginning with an understanding of the premise of regression therapy, then moving on to actual experiences of healing through the case studies of some of my clients, and finally ending with lessons gained and discoveries made over the journey. The guidance of my spiritual gurus has been paramount in awakening the inner wisdom.

The greatest lesson I have learned so far—and reasserted through the healing journey of almost every client—is how little we really know. It is in the light of this realisation that I welcome you to read this book.

Dr Natwar Sharma
India, 2020

I
PREMISES

The Physical—and Beyond

The body never lies. *But the truth is rarely limited to the physical.*

When I am approached by clients with their physical ailments, I tell them and, more importantly, I remind myself that the manifesting issue is but the tip of the iceberg. The solution lies in exploring the mountain underneath. I have also observed that when a person is suffering from multiple health issues, usually there is a single underlying cause that triggers the problems—like a strike in a game of bowling. You aim at the right spot, or precisely at just one pin, and bingo! All the pins are knocked off, and you have pocketed a strike. Similarly, such a single underlying cause usually surfaces during the course of regression therapy, and this becomes the key to resolving all the health issues of the client. In most cases, the cause is not restricted to the physical body.

Being trained as a mainstream doctor, my mind was fixed on the process of treatment: etiology, pathogenesis, diagnosis, prognosis and prescription. I could think only in one direction, and specialisation in this field appeared to me like the classic case of trying to get the whole vision of the forest with a close-up of just one tree! What made me deviate from tradition was the realisation that mainstream medicine does not really address all the nuances of the disease. Treatment and medication are purely symptom-based, and diagnosis of the disease focusses on either genetic or environmental factors. In some exceptional cases, the disease is diagnosed as idiopathic, because we have no clue about the cause.

Even as we are able to arrive at an accurate diagnosis from the symptoms, I am intrigued by the variety of ways and the grades in which the same disease can manifest in different individuals. For example, dengue can manifest in different grades. So, while one person is mildly affected by the disease, it can be fatal for another. Similarly, while there may be a common criterion to diagnose migraine—like the manifestation of three of the five basic symptoms—it can manifest in different degrees in different individuals, or even in the same individual in different degrees at different points in time.

Very soon, and contrary to my training, I had the inkling that every disease was unique to the individual—that there was something unique to each individual that acts as a trigger for the disorder or disease to manifest the way it does. My opening to the regression technique of healing turned my hunch into conviction.

Try this as an experiment: observe your physical body during various activities. For example, note the reactions in your body while watching an emotionally charged programme on television, especially horror shows or thrillers. Your muscles may contract without your knowledge, and your heart may pulsate at a faster rate. These somatic charges in the body, directly or indirectly determine the level of stress you experience during the day. Similarly, uttering a word or a phrase or a sentence charged with an emotion produces a physical charge in the body. You may feel tightness or heaviness, weakness or pain or a tingling sensation in some part of the body while saying, 'I am feeling scared.' Repeat this experiment with different sentences conveying positive and negative emotions, and see what reactions they produce in the body. You may be amazed at what you observe and feel.

It is important here to note the difference between feeling and emotion. For example, I may feel left out or not included in a particular situation, but what sort of emotion does this feeling generate? As an adult, I may be sad that I was not included. As a child, I may be angry at my parents for leaving me out of some talk or activity, or I may even be guilty because I did not do what I was supposed to do and, as a result, I automatically missed being a part of something. Generally, I may have a sense of helplessness, and sometimes, I may even experience a mixture of emotions. Thus, *one* situation can produce a cocktail of emotions, which can be debilitating, when suppressed for long. Here, the length of time is not restricted to the present, for, isn't the present life but a fragment in the continuity of existence?

My clients include people who belong to faiths that do not propagate the idea of reincarnation, and most of them initially don't believe in past lives. Yet, when for whatsoever reason they come to me and show interest in regression, I tell them to keep their minds open and explore, whether they believe or not. I tell them plainly, 'Just because you believe something exists, doesn't mean you can prove it. And just because you believe something doesn't exist, doesn't mean you are right. Go with the flow and see what your mind is waiting to show you.'

Then, as they go through a session and gain an insight into their past, they automatically start linking it with their present. When they understand for themselves how intrinsically the patterns are connected and how changes occur in their present lives, they start believing in the idea of reincarnation after that.

There are also cases where clients don't believe what they see; they feel they've imagined it. But when they start establishing connections between their past and present by themselves, when they start acknowledging certain patterns ruling their lives, when they start seeing positive changes, and when the healing seeps in, they say, 'Oh yes, this cannot be denied. I have been suffering from this problem for decades, and now within ten days, I see a huge change in myself! How can this be possible?'

I am inclined to think that the very fact that clients from different faiths come to me for therapy establishes their belief in reincarnation, although they may not immediately admit it. Deep down, they have a belief, but the mental conditioning from childhood that 'there is no past life' prevents them from being open to exploring. Deep down they *know* that the soul exists and that it is on an infinite journey, but they take time and experience to acknowledge it.

In some cases, even when they go through regression and see the changes that follow, they still don't believe. They feel it is merely their imagination that led to catharsis and helped them. And I am perfectly fine with that, for, ultimately, as a doctor and therapist, all that matters to me is my patients' and clients' healing. 'Are you feeling better? Perfect. You still don't believe in past lives? That's okay, too.'

Interestingly, some of my clients belonging to faiths who do not believe in reincarnation have actually confided in me that even their scriptures talk about the eternal existence of the soul through life afterlife. For example, a man from the Middle East came to me once and said, 'I need help. I believe in past life. It exists in my religion, in our holy scriptures.'

No matter what we choose to think or believe, in essence, we *are* souls. And the second commonality is that we are human beings as a species. That we are born with different skin colours and just because we are conditioned religiously from childhood in a different way, it doesn't mean we are different from each other. We share similar patterns of lives, both past and present. There is nothing unique; it's all the same.

Let's look at the topic of reincarnation from the viewpoint of evolution. Most of the theories indicate genetic mutation or cellular division—from the unicellular to the multicellular—through space and time. If such a mutation can happen between different species, I am inclined to believe in its occurrence *within* the species—*in each unit of the same species*. Setting aside its esoteric and mystical connotation, and plainly viewing it through the glass of science, I see reincarnation as nothing but a way of evolution of the individual soul. Whether it facilitates evolution beyond the human existence—if at all further evolution is possible—is an answer that I will save for my readers to infer from this book.

It may be interesting to observe the human body after death, from a clinical perspective, and compare it with when the person was alive. A striking difference that may be evident, not just to somebody from a medical background but even to a layman, is the change in energy levels. Someone familiar with the science of aura-reading may be able to note the change in the aura of the human body after death.

Today, tons of data is transferred through wireless modes. We cannot see the data which is transmitted, because it is not physical. Still, we can transmit and access the information: *subtle energy is transported by subtle means.* Research in the fields of psychology and parapsychology indicate that such a subtle transfer of energy is possible not just through space but even through time—that information, or memory, from one lifetime can be transferred to another lifetime.

In his research on reincarnation, Dr Ian Stevenson came across children with past-life memories: he was able to trace the cause of some of their physical features such as birthmarks and certain physical defects to such impressions of the past. In my own experience as a paediatrician and regression therapist, I found that some children who were born with a hole in their heart, had, in fact, died in a previous life with a bullet in their heart. They were shot at, and they carried the memory of that hole in the heart into their present life. Similarly, one of my clients came in with a history of Stroke's Adam Syndrome—where the heart suddenly stops beating and the person loses consciousness. Through regression, we discovered that the syndrome was a physical manifestation of the client's traumatic memory of being stabbed in the heart in her past life. The lady recovered as she began to understand what was really manifesting.

In the light of these evidences, I infer that when the life force—which I choose to call 'soul' for the lack of any other familiar terminology—leaves the body at the time of death, it carries an energy domain, like a big invisible network, consisting of impressions of the past life. This subtle body of information influences the genetic makeup of the new physical body—its genes and chromosomes. I find this form of energy transfer quite amazing, and I like to term it as 'information packed in vibration', or 'energy in motion'—e-motion.

The physical manifestation of diseases in our present life can be linked to such cellular memories from the past, including even childhood or early stages of our present life—especially when the stored memories are negative or traumatic. When we don't let out these e-motions, they get trapped or stored in a particular body part. Eventually, this energy disturbance starts influencing the body structure—the cells and the tissues—leading to diseases and disorders. I would like to coin a new terminology for this pattern—Psycho-cyto-pathology. It describes how the psyche, our feelings, emotions and thoughts, produce disease (pathos) in the cell (cyto).

Most diseases, especially chronic ailments, are psychosomatic in nature. For example, a chronic frozen shoulder could most likely be the physical manifestation of a traumatic memory of an accident in the past that is stored over a period of time in the bones, muscles, cartilage and ligaments of the body.

Sometimes, the manifestation of such an energy disturbance at the molecular level is immediate, while in other cases, it takes longer for the disorder to develop in the physical body. Ailments like hypertension and diabetes that manifest later in life are a result of years of emotionally abusing our system, in addition to the negative emotions that percolate from childhood into adult life. Hence, it is in the interest of our health and well-being to deal with our emotions at an early stage in our life. We can simply blow away the tender shoot as soon as it sprouts out of the soil, but as it grows into a strong, sturdy tree, we need an axe or a machine to bring it down. Moreover, if we only cut at the surface, the tree is sure to grow from the roots again under suitable conditions. Addressing our emotional issues is like preventive medicine: we deal with the issue when it is still tender and release the emotion from our system before it can manifest as a physical ailment or disease. Instead of suppressing the symptoms, we deal with the roots—the triggers of the symptoms.

We need to understand that the disease usually starts in the mind—our thoughts influence our emotions. Thoughts have a deeper consequence than actual action because the physical body is superficial and merely the manifesting layer of all that lies covered underneath. This understanding will help us deal with our overall health: *if our thoughts can make us fall sick, they can also help us heal.*

The Scope of Regression Therapy
Vis-à-Vis Mainstream Medicine

The body can be a true guide to what lies beyond. In most cases where the body does not manifest any malfunction or disorder, I am inclined to believe that the person's health is largely sound and whatever discomfort he may be experiencing in his overall well-being can possibly be resolved with ongoing medication. But sometimes it is purely psychological without any somatic manifestations and disturbs an individual's life. Usually, when people approach me for regression out of fun or to satisfy their curiosity, I say 'No', politely, but firmly.

Regression is a serious, life-changing business. An awareness and responsibility of this fact is what I solicit from all my clients going through the therapy. I humbly state that my experience as a mainstream physician grants me the advantage of understanding the disease in its totality, from diagnosis to prognosis. Unless I find evidence and intuitively feel that the person needs to heal through regression, I do not recommend it.

I recollect one of my first few cases of regression, where my client, Akshara, was suffering from a very rare disorder of the red blood cells. The information about her past that emerged through regression bowled me over. I was at a loss about connecting this information about my client's past with what was manifesting in her present. I was almost going to give up on the case and even reconsider my prospects as a therapist when intuition took over rationality. I began to see pieces of the puzzle falling into place, clearly. But then I began to reconsider my status as a mainstream physician. While I had answers to my client's current situation, I questioned the very purpose of the time and effort I had spent in studying medicine. I received answers that were life-changing.

Akshara's case made me realise that books cannot really teach us everything, unless we convert the knowledge in them into an experience of our own. Openness is the key. If we are conditioned from the beginning about anything or anyone and start analysing them as right or wrong, we miss going with the flow. The mind is a beautiful tool—it unwinds slowly, and once we allow it to unwind totally, we may have this eureka moment: 'Aha, now it all matches!' The answer simply emerges—as it happened with me in Akshara's case.

The greater realisation, which later progressed into conviction, was of the fact that my studying medicine with all its nuances had not been a waste of time and effort. On the contrary, if I didn't know the pathogenesis of a manifesting disease, I would not have been able to link the rather 'dry' piece of information from my client's past life to her unusual disease in the present. That is why I feel it is advantageous for the therapist—even if he or she is not an adroit physician—to have at least basic knowledge of medical science to understand the functioning of the human body, how diseases come into being and the nature of the pathogenesis. With a basic background and understanding of pathologies and medical conditions, therapists can probe deeper and derive a comprehensive knowledge of the client's symptoms and manifestations leading to successful diagnosis and cure. In regression therapy, one has to make the connection between the disease and the cause to use the clues as metaphors from the past to heal in the present. And such perception and understanding are expected on the part of both the therapist and the client, to facilitate better healing.

According to my experience, this link between the past and the present in the form of metaphors is the premise on which healing occurs through regression. And this is the central theme of most of the cases that have been presented in this book. In the chapters that follow, we will see how healing and recovery take place as clients begin to observe, experience and learn from the repetitive patterns of past and present lives. The case studies reveal the etiopathology of certain diseases that cannot be explained by mainstream medicine. This premise also opens us to a new facet of regression—which needs further exploration and research—and to its scope as a healing technique in the light of mainstream medicine.

——

While most chronic conditions and ailments have a potential cure in regression therapy, acute disorders and diseases are better handled by mainstream medicine. For example, many people come to me with kidney failure that ideally calls for dialysis or transplant. They ask me to help them out of such painful situations with a cure. Now, the fact is that kidney cells do not regenerate. Once those cells are dead, they are dead.

So, I clearly and gently explain to my patients: 'A fire has destroyed the forest; the trees that are burnt won't come back. But we can at least find out the source of the fire: where did it come from? If we can identify the source, in the future we may be able to control the fire from burning the remaining trees in the forest.'

Kidney ailments are mostly progressive: they go on and on, slowly bringing up the level of creatinine in the body. Through regression, there is a possibility of stopping that progression or recurrence and save the tissues and cells that are still leftover.

And how does this happen? Well, regression gives us the understanding of an insight into our thought process and our emotions that are majorly fuelling the disease. As we begin to understand that we, ourselves, have invited this disease, we can accept the present situation, which in turn, makes us willing and open to whatever needs to be done to take care of the remaining organ. So, we shift from a defeatist attitude to one that is embracing: 'All right, if I need to go through dialysis or a transplant, so be it.'

We are fortunate to be in an era where we have innovative methods, aided by technology, which help us live and add quality to life. Wisdom lies in using them for this purpose, and there is certainly no harm in doing so.

So far, I haven't come across any research-based evidence which shows that such cases, like chronic renal failure or damage to the brain due to a stroke, can be cured and cells regenerated. But in the case of allergic skin disorders, like eczema or psoriasis, in addition to diet and lifestyle changes, doctors often recommend hypnotherapy, mindful practices and visualisation to address the underlying psychological stress that is strongly linked to the manifestation of these skin conditions. The connection between the mind and body is used to cure this disorder. The scope of regression extends, but is not limited to such chronic cases.

Regression therapy also works as an excellent alternative treatment for most mental and psychological disorders. The most significant edge that this therapy has over conventional methods is that instead of suppressing the symptoms it can trace their origin and subsequently eliminated them from the roots. At the same time, when people suffering from depression approach me, I don't stop their medicines immediately, because these antidepressants are sometimes helpful in acute cases where you need to calm down the patient first to start the treatment.

Moreover, stopping these medicines abruptly would affect the neuro-transmitters of the body and thus can manifest as withdrawal symptoms and side-effects in the patient. Similarly, in the case of autoimmune diseases, the symptoms may suddenly flare up and cannot be handled unless you treat them with steroids and other anti-inflammatory medicines. As the symptoms recede, you can deal with the patient through this therapy, which usually involves a series of sessions over a period of time. When the person begins to understand the reason for his disorder and his physical symptoms start improving, the medicines can be tapered off under medical supervision.

—-—

As my clients' vision opens to their past, my treatment plan becomes clearer. As there is a definite bridge between mainstream medicine and regression therapy, I see a huge scope for the integration of these modalities of treatment, one conventional and the other non-conventional. I request my readers to read with an open mind, to understand that there is so much beyond what is obvious. I also solicit the willingness and openness of my medical brotherhood to view the case studies presented in this book as subject matter for further research and study in this revolutionary area of health and medicine. Believe it or not, much of our healing depends on *us*—and that forms the basis of the next chapter.

The Nature and Time of Healing

'Well begun is half done'—the significance of the intent and faith behind the action, rather than the action itself, strikes me as the underlying meaning of this saying by Aristotle. I am inclined to believe in its truth even in the process of healing, irrespective of the mode of treatment or medication. Coincidentally, the term 'catharsis' was also used for the first time by Aristotle in one of his works as a metaphor. He compared the effects of tragedy on a spectator's mind to the effect of a cathartic on the body.

In medicine, a cathartic is a substance that accelerates defecation in the body. In a layman's terms, it helps in cleansing the body of toxic or impure elements. I was excited to discover that the word 'catharsis' also means 'purification' or 'cleansing'—but of e-motions that are mostly negative. Needless to say, most of the healing in regression therapy happens through catharsis during the integration of past and present lives. What a cathartic does to the physical body made up of cells and tissues, mental and emotional catharsis does to the subtle body of past impressions and information.

During the therapy, catharsis may not always happen by way of crying; sometimes the client may experience catharsis even by laughing heartily. There are other instances, too, where the experience of love or gratitude makes one cry more than pain and suffering. Whether my clients cry or laugh, what concerns me as a therapist is their comprehensive recovery—and with this primary motive, I deal with each and every nuance of the therapy.

Often, deep experiences come within the fold of regression, making one wonder about the question of existence beyond the physical. In many cases during regression, after the soul leaves the body at the end of a lifetime, it usually goes through a period of 'rest' during which it meets other souls, who are mostly its ancestors or guides who help in choosing its next course of existence. These rest periods, constituting interactions with higher beings or enlightened souls, can be full of wisdom and higher learning for the client in question, through the understanding and experience of which they may choose to transform and heal. Each session has the potential to teach great lessons, and, to facilitate healing through such learning, I go with whatever is comfortable to my client. If they choose to dwell between lifetimes and be guided by other souls, so be it. Irrespective of whether it appeals to everybody, this book throws light on healing through such a 360-degree understanding of the purpose of human existence.

—-—

At the onset of therapy, my client and I usually agree on the problem we want to address through regression. Such clarity is important because, while we may face multiple problems, only one or a few may actually be bothering or adversely affecting daily existence. Moreover, there may be a single underlying cause behind the manifesting issues we are not consciously aware of. Sometimes, a single lifetime may be the key to many of our manifesting and underlying issues in the present. Tapping into that particular lifetime is like a drop that refines the entire ocean. So, we begin by identifying the issue that we want to address and, as the sessions evolve with my client, often what was not apparent comes to light. As soon as I see clarity regarding the cause of the manifesting problem—both in myself and my client—I close the session after the integration.

Healing, in regression, mostly happens through integration after catharsis. I prefer calling it reintegration because, in essence and origin, we are integrated beings. When we do not take charge of our lives, we tend to breakdown and disintegrate, losing our energies or a part of ourselves. Through regression when we understand the situation as it is, we are able to let go of the emotion that is holding us back, retrieve our lost part or parts, and become whole again. It is also in this sense that regression works as a holistic therapy.

Sometimes, a client is not ready and willing to face the experience that comes in the fold of regression. Healing is largely dependent on the client's willingness to face his past and the different facets of himself that he may probably be exposed to through this therapy. The experience has a lot of wisdom and understanding attached to it. Such experiences may change the perception of how we look at ourselves and the world around us. Recovery through this therapy is neither difficult nor easy because it involves the client's willing participation. After all, it takes two to tango! If the person is aware and consciously cooperates, then the healing is much faster. This experience was well-articulated by one of my clients who came to me with multiple issues and went through a fascinating journey of overall recovery.

There is a certain intellectual process that occurs during your healing. It is not that you come out of a regression session and your body immediately accepts whatever has happened and feels all fine—no. You also have to work with your conscious mind to heal your body, but the process is accelerated. Earlier, what would happen is that when there is a trigger of a memory of the past in the present, it would manifest as a disorder or disease in your body. Your mind may not accept it and you are likely to crib and deny the situation. *Why is this happening to me?* But because of all that transpires in these sessions, the mind and the body begin a dance—they tango in tandem. A lot of the work happens during the break that the therapist gives between sessions, and the healing manifests as considerable changes in your physical and mental being. There is a synthesis of all the elements—of the mind and body, of the past and present, of wisdom and understanding.

Let me elucidate this. Normally, after a session, clients mostly report significant changes in their patterns of thinking and behaving, which occur spontaneously and automatically. However, they may be tested on certain tendencies that are quite strong, through situations that push them to their threshold of tolerance and it is likely that they may slip and repeat the past mistakes. But that is where the role of the conscious mind or the individual will come into play, saying, 'Well, I have made this mistake in the past, and I know the consequences. I don't want to repeat it and trouble or punish myself. I will take charge of my life, and I will not let this happen again.' Here, based on the knowledge of the past, we have to make a conscious effort by applying our will to change.

Thus, part of the healing happens spontaneously, and for the rest, we have to pedal a little. In this process, a new neuro pathway develops; the brain rewires to integrate the change with our being. Then the question of applying the will does not arise, for then it becomes natural. So, this brain rewiring is very important for complete recovery, which may ideally take place over three to six months after the session or sessions. As my responsible client asserts above, this gap between sessions is quite significant where much of the healing manifests. At the same time, it also gives room for follow-ups and reviews that are vital to the complete closure of the client's issue.

It is likely that the person may feel fine immediately after one session, but only a review can actually tell the degree or depth of recovery. In my experience, I have found that certain disorders like obesity, are usually triggered by multiple emotional or energy blocks over multiple lifetimes, which call for healing through multiple layers. Each follow-up session with the client may reveal a new layer or a new facet of the manifesting issue, and until all facets are dealt with, the disorder may persist in some way or other. Improvement in the physical symptoms—determined by blood test reports, a scan or an X-ray at the end of six months after the last session—is a trusted way to have a clear idea of the extent of recovery.

Some clients report a total recovery after one session, while some others heal over a series of sessions. This time period of healing varies from person to person. I have observed that it mostly depends upon the depth of the imprint that a particular incident leaves on the subtle make-up of the individual. The faster the cellular memories wane, the faster is the recovery from the disease.

While recovery can be measured in terms of improvement in the physical symptoms and subtly through a sense of balance and harmony in the person's emotional and mental capacities, whether we can ascribe a uniform pattern or time of healing for each disease or disorder is a question that can be answered only through well-documented regression sessions conducted scientifically and thoroughly with the help of proper research methodologies over a period of time.

Clearly, healing through regression requires the client's cooperation and willingness to release and let go of traumatic memories of the past; hence, to state that, as a therapist, I cure my clients would be sheer arrogance. The mind is the real healer, with huge potential that is tapped during regression. My clients heal themselves; I *only* facilitate. All credit goes to the client's mind for the healing, and the therapist is just a guide in the process. *The mind is a double-edged sword: if it can produce a disease, it can also heal.*

II

CASE STUDIES

A Sense of Insecurity
One Common Cause for Several Psychosomatic Conditions

When a person feels a lack of support in the family or in professional and social circles, it can lead to many complications, affecting the well-being of the individual. The most severe impact is at the psychological level with the person feeling lonely and very desolate. Research on the connection between body and mind, reveals that several disorders and diseases arise from this psychosomatic condition or feeling of desolation.

Imagine a scenario where the soldiers of our physical system, the white blood corpuscles, turn against the body. Our protectors turn into the ones who harm us. Here are a few cases where this suppressed emotion of being let down by one's own kith and kin becomes a metaphor for the clients' present physical issues.

—

A forty-three-year-old man, Anand, who suffered from severe leg pain and weakness, was unable to walk without crutches. Extensive medical investigations led to the diagnosis of fibromyalgia, which is a disorder characterised by chronic musculoskeletal pain that is often accompanied by sleep, fatigue, memory and mood issues. The symptoms of this disorder mostly appear after a physical trauma or significant mental stress, and its cause is generally associated with psychological, genetic, neurological and environmental factors. While a variety of medications can control the symptoms, there is no established cure for fibromyalgia in mainstream medicine. As this disorder got worse, Anand was scared and insecure about his family and future.

I clearly remember the day he walked into my clinic on crutches. With sad and gloomy eyes, he seemed to lack confidence and appeared like someone in a lot of pain and despair. As I started noting his history, he broke down into tears.

> Anand: Almost a year ago, I developed pain in both my feet, the intensity of which gradually started progressing. Now the pain has increased to such an extent that if I take more than ten to fifteen steps, it gets severe and I cannot walk anymore. That's when I have to use my crutches. The calf muscles of both my legs feel very tight and compressed. Heel pads are not working any more, and I have been experiencing numbness in three of my toes since the last five months.
>
> The worst part is that I am unable to go to office since the last three months and I have been working from home. My boss has given me one more month to join back. Otherwise, I will lose my job. I feel very helpless and distracted because of which I am unable to focus on my work. I have a ten-year-old daughter. I feel so insecure. I feel helpless. I'm useless. I'm so angry at myself.

As I probed deeper into his personal life, he mentioned that he had a very bad relationship with his younger brother.

> Anand: My younger brother is quite cunning and my mother supports him. I love my mother a lot but she has never reciprocated in the same way. Ten years ago, when I lost my job and didn't have anything in my hands, I had to depend on my younger brother and my father for monetary support. It didn't go well at all.

Soon after this, we met again for his first session of regression. As he lay on the recliner in my clinic, I began by asking him a few questions.

Me: Okay. Now tell me, what do your feet mean to you?

Anand: My feet help me in moving around—and in earning money. They are a very important part of my body; I'm dependent on them.

This statement from my client indicated self-dependency. Next, I asked him what his painful feet meant to him.

Anand: It means dependency; I have to be dependent. I feel miserable, helpless and angry as I hate being dependent on anybody. The worst part is when people pity me.

At this juncture, Anand interrupted saying the pain in his feet was increasing. This was reassuring to me because I knew his body had started reacting. We were on the right track.

Anand: Look at my feet … they are blue, swollen and lifeless.

Though not very convincing, I couldn't help but notice a blue hue around his feet. My intuition guided me to deduce that he was ready for regression. I asked my client to close his eyes, and I began to give him suggestions that would intensify the emotions that he felt along with the pain that was manifesting. Very easily and quickly, Anand regressed into a past life.

Anand: I see a beggar sitting under a tree. It's me … I am wearing a dirty dhoti, and a dirty vest with multiple holes in it. I am leaning against something and my legs are slightly spread. I am only skin and bones. My legs feel so lifeless that I can't even move them. My hair looks dirty and unkempt; my skin also looks the same. I have tanned under the sun; I look dark. I look much older than I am. I am emaciated. People are passing by, but no one wants to look at me. They are just ignoring me and walking away as if I don't exist. How can one human being treat another so badly? It's terrible. I notice a lady passing by and when she sees me, she covers her nose with her sari, making me realise I am probably stinking, but I can't smell it.

At this, my client began to cry in this deep trance, completely identifying himself with this personality.

> Anand: My heart is so heavy, filled with sadness. It is as if there is a huge stone on my heart. My whole body feels really heavy. I'm thirsty and hungry, but I have no energy to stand up. I have been trying to get up, but every time I do, I feel dizzy. I have been trying to pick myself up for a while and now I finally feel like giving up. I just want to die; I'm waiting for death. Death will be a big relief.

With a simple suggestion to move to the next significant moment, Anand moved to the time of his death in that lifetime.

> Anand: I am seeing darkness alternating with light, as if I'm losing consciousness and gaining it again, and finally everything is dark. I think I am there ... I can see my body under a tree, leaning against a dirty trash bag on the street. My soul feels relieved, but I also feel very sad, looking at my body stuck there and unable to move. My body is just a bundle of bones. Finally, I see two men coming and even they close their nose as they approach me. I must be stinking very badly ... These two men put me on a rickshaw and fully cover my body with the dirty clothes. I am being taken away. I feel a deep sense of relief, but there is also a question as to why I had to go through such a horrible life, such a horrible death. I vaguely remember my family, but it's not clear.

At this juncture, I give him a suggestion to move back in time when he was with his family. Anand regressed further back in that lifetime.

> Anand: I am a thirty-year-old man wearing a dhoti and kurta. I have a turban on my head. It's a big house with wooden pillars and tiled roof. It looks like a village setting. I'm wearing leather footwear. I am well-built and good-looking. When I walk on the streets of the village, people respect me; they salute me. I think I am the head of the village, and I carry a kind of pride with me that people like me. It feels like the early 20th century. Somewhere in the south of India, perhaps in Karnataka...

I reach home. I see an old man, about sixty years old. I think he is my father. He is thin and frail-looking and is sitting on a couch. Our house has a big central courtyard, and there are many rooms, all big-sized. There are many servants at home. I have a big family: two brothers and one sister, all married. The sister's husband also lives with us. I am the eldest. My wife is a pious and beautiful lady and I have two young daughters, eight- and six-year-old. They are very happy to see me.

Everything looks fine, but I get a strange feeling from my brothers who seem to carry a fake smile. I feel as if something is happening in the background, something is happening behind me. I see my mother but I sense some sort of indifference in her too. When my daughters come running to hug me, it takes away this negative feeling. And when I step out of the house, I feel much better because people genuinely love me for my straightforwardness, honesty, and helpful nature. I do not take it when people try to manipulate me.

There was a pause. It gave me the opportunity to intervene and give a suggestion, prompting Anand to go deeper to explore the root cause behind the negativity he sensed in his brothers' demeanour.

Anand: My father was the head of the village and I took over from him at the age of twenty-five, in front of the whole village. As a child, I saw my father taking decisions slowly and being very tolerant of the villagers' misdoings. He allowed people to manipulate things. Growing up, I thought I would not give room for this. After I took charge, I really did not allow such things to happen. I took decisions quickly, unlike my father, and I put pressure on people to get work done faster. My father advises me to slow down, but I don't listen to him. My brothers, who don't seem to really like me, behave nicely superficially. They start feeding negative things about me to my father. I am adamant and I don't listen to my father. I have brought growth to the village and people respect me, not out of fear but out of love. The wrongdoers are definitely scared of me. I notice that my father is distancing himself from me. He used to be so close to me.

I see another old man—my father-in-law—who has come to see me. We are near a big farmland. He is advising me to be careful and have the property divided properly. He senses that my brothers may harm me. I get very angry and upset with him and insult him in front of the whole village, telling him that it's none of his business to interfere in our family matters, and that we are a wonderfully united family and my brothers cannot cheat me. My father-in-law is offended and angry, but he doesn't have the courage to speak in front of me and silently walks away.

I gently suggested that he move forward to the next significant moment to understand what had gone wrong.

Anand: I am around forty years of age. I am entering the house one evening and I see my brother, sister and brother-in-law standing at the entrance of the house. I also see my father sitting on the cot in a corner. I'm surprised to see them all waiting at the entrance in this manner, and ask my father what the issue is. In reply, he asks me to leave the house with my belongings. I am completely shocked to hear this and I have no words to utter. My brother urges, 'Leave now. Can't you hear what father just said?' I feel completely abandoned. I begin to have severe pain in my chest, as if a dagger has been thrust in my heart. I feel betrayed and abandoned.

I feel offended at being thrown out of my own house. I decide not to take anything and am only accompanied by my wife and kids. My wife suggests we go to her father's house, but I think otherwise and decide to go to a place where nobody knows us, because I don't want my family's pride to be destroyed. As we are walking out of the house, the villagers who know me, wish me well. I see tears in their eyes: they don't want me to go. But I also see people who are happy that I am leaving.

We keep walking until it is very dark and decide to rest under a tree. I tell my wife that I want to go back and ask my father and brother why they did this. But my wife doesn't let me go; she is not in favour of the idea. I feel sad for my kids, who are asleep and hungry.

When my wife too falls asleep, I decide to go back to the village to confront my family. As I reach home, I am stopped by two men. They are none other than my own brothers, who do not allow me to enter the house. I feel even more humiliated, dejected and angry. My whole body is burning in anger and I feel like crying. I can't even talk to my own father! I feel like committing suicide.

I walk back to the same spot where I had left my wife and daughters, but to my surprise, I find them missing. I feel heartbroken. A beggar nearby conveys a message from my wife: she had asked me to take care of myself and said that she was going to her father's place with our daughters. I begin to cry, I knew this would happen. My wife is a very sensible lady. She gave me the option of going to her father's place for our children's safety, but because I could not drop my pride, I did not agree. I'm sure she has taken this decision for the safety of our daughters, because she knows I am adamant.

A part of me feels relieved that at least my daughters and wife are safe. I decide to go to a new place to start a new life, work hard, and then bring back my family. But I also have this fear that I don't have any skills to do any work; all I did in the village was to give orders and have people obey my orders.

Finally, I move to a bigger town where I see lots of people. I begin to work by lifting gunny bags and loading them into bullock carts. At the end of the day, I earn a pittance, which is sufficient only to fill my stomach. I feel so miserable thinking that if it continues the same way, I may never be able to get my family back. So, I decide to work longer. I eat less so that I'm able to save money to bring my family back. A few months pass by in this manner. I become weaker and I'm not able to physically perform well at work.

One day, as I carry out the task of loading the gunny bags, I feel as if my feet are sinking into the ground. I push myself. Every step feels so heavy. Suddenly, I collapse. I hear a crack; I have hurt my leg....

On the recliner, in my clinic, Anand actually winced in pain trying to touch his ankle.

Anand: It feels like a bad injury. My right ankle has twisted and I'm not able to get up. I'm dragging myself to a corner, feeling shy and conscious. My foot seems to be broken. What will I do now? I can't carry the load to earn money to fill my own stomach. I wait for the foot to heal, for the pain to relieve, but it is not getting any better. This is just an add-on to the existing weakness in my legs, and I was just pushing myself too hard.

As the days pass by, I resort to begging. I sit near the temple to beg. It is so humiliating that I cover my face, so that no one recognises me. I don't feel like eating, but the pang of hunger is very strong. I recollect those days when, on special occasions, I would feed the whole village. All my strength and pride as a zamindar seems hollow. I feel I will never see my family again. I feel I have lost everything. I have lost my courage, my pride, and my confidence. I have lost my own self.

I look ugly, dirty and dark. I can't walk without a walking stick, which I have made out of a tree branch. My legs have become thin and weak. I can see the veins. My neck hurts badly. My whole body is in pain. My hands feel numb. I hate looking at my own body.

I deeply regret what happened. I feel the villagers tricked me because I wanted to bring discipline, honesty and prosperity to everyone. I don't know where I went wrong; how could I have done things differently? I hate manipulation. I don't know what I did to deserve this kind of life? I feel anger towards God. I am just waiting for death.

After a brief pause, Anand moved again to the time when his soul is watching his dead body.

Anand: I was just a toy at their disposal ...

He cried bitterly for a minute. I waited.

Anand: I didn't expect this from my father. I always thought he would support me. I feel I am not his son. I did not have sons and that is the reason he listens to my younger brother.

I was surprised to hear when he said, "I am not his son." I asked Anand what made him feel so. He said it was not clear but he kind of grew up with that feeling. With a simple suggestion, I asked him to go back in time to the moment where he would be able to get more clarity about his parents.

> Anand: I am a four-year-old boy with hardly any clothes on my body. I am wearing torn shorts. I am hungry and thirsty. I seem to be looking for my parents who have left me. I don't know why, but I think there was not enough food and we were starving. I look very thin and frail. I remember two days ago when my thin and frail mother and father were starving to feed me.

This was quite intriguing. I gently prodded Anand to recollect, if he could, the reason for his parents leaving him.

> Anand: We are living in a shanty made of bamboo sticks. My father and mother do labour work, and when they don't get work, they beg. One evening, I see my father caring a lot for me and showing much affection. He is hugging and telling me that things will be fine, that I should be strong and take care of myself.
>
> Next morning, as I wake up, I find both my parents missing; they seem to have abandoned me. I had sensed something wrong the previous night, when my father was comforting me, for he had never lavished so much affection in that manner ever before. I had slept peacefully, but when I woke up, I found my world had come to an end. There is an old man nearby, who tells me that my parents had sold themselves as slaves. I don't understand: How can they leave me?
>
> I am just roaming around aimlessly. That's when the Zamindar finds me and takes me to his home. He gives me clothes to wear and food to eat. He then declares to the village that I am his son. I feel very happy that I am being loved and I am well taken care of. After a few years, my father has his biological children, and we are all living happily.

Anand paused yet again.

Anand: I am happy that at least my wife took the wise decision to take the children to her father.

Me: Do you feel any anger towards your father or brothers?

Anand: I have no anger towards father because I know he's a good man. He was manipulated by my brothers.

Me: Did you have a choice? Could you have handled the circumstances differently?

Anand: I was very adamant and arrogant. My brothers were insecure; they felt that I would take away everything. But I had no intention to cheat my brothers. I was not greedy and that's why I left home without taking anything. My arrogance was stronger than my wisdom. I should have taken my share. I should have had the humility to accept what rightfully belonged to me. Because of my arrogance, not only did I suffer, but I made my family suffer too. Humility is a very important lesson of this life.

But why did I choose a life like this, where I was abandoned even as a small child and then later had to experience betrayal from my own family members again?

At this point, I chose to take him back in time, as his soul had already left the body in that life. I gave him the suggestion to go back to yet another lifetime to understand the *karma* he had created in the past, because his soul chose to go through abandonment and betrayal. Anand regressed further to a time before his life as the Zamindar.

Anand: I see myself as a soldier, probably German. I am under training and I can see lots of other soldiers like me are training very hard. We have a hound that we have to feed and train and take care of. We run faster and faster with every passing day, with very tough training. We kill brutally, without feelings or emotions. If we don't speed up every day, we don't get our meal. We finish the assigned task to get our meal. Speed is very important.

The dog has become a very good friend and that's the only company at night. One day, I am completely shocked when our commander gives us the order to kill the dog. For a moment, I am unable to react but I have no choice, and I take out the dagger and stab the dog under its ear. I feel I have become numb—no feelings, no emotions, just like a mechanical robot. I feel dead from inside. We keep moving from one place to another, and our success is counted by the number of people we kill, and the speed with which we accomplish our jobs. Our commander doesn't appreciate easily.

One night, we are suddenly attacked. I can see Polish soldiers killing many of us. I am stabbed in my left arm, and I don't want to die. I try to strike a deal with the commander of the Polish army so that they spare my life. I disclose to them the whereabouts of the other German soldiers in hiding. I escape and move on to live a mediocre life till the age of sixty. But the guilt that I traded my friends to save my own life never left me.

This was a revelation to me as well as my client. I guided him in making a connection between the two lives: that of the zamindar betrayed by his family in South India, and the German soldier who had betrayed his fellow soldiers. It was clear that his act of betraying his fellow soldiers was the *karma* responsible for all that he had to undergo in his life as the zamindar. Based on these past lives, I asked him if he could see similarities or patterns in his current life.

Anand: Yes. From the life of a zamindar I have carried the memory of pain in my feet, legs, neck and body, and the numbness in my hands along with insecurity and fear of not being able to take care of my family members. I seem to have carried even the arrogance that I can discipline anyone!

From the soldier's life, I have carried the memory of the belief that I can do a lot of work at top speed. In the process, sometimes, I become so numb, not respecting the feelings and emotions of my subordinates at work.

Reliving those moments of the past intensified his feeling of a lack of support in the present—his inability to support his family and the lack of support from his siblings. The metaphor also reflected in the present life—his legs that were meant to support him, had given way and he had to seek the aid of crutches instead.

After he had made these connections, I gave Anand a suggestion to move back in time in his present life when his fear and insecurity were triggered for the first time.

> Anand: I am thirty-three year old. My boss calls me and tells me that I am fired. I'm not completely sure of the reason; the boss is not saying anything clearly. I feel so bad and angry to receive this kind of treatment from my boss after working so hard, and even completing one year's project in just three months! I am sitting at my desk in the office, shutting down my computer, and my mind is filled with thoughts about the loan I have taken and the EMI I have to pay. My child is quite young and I wonder how I'll sustain my family.
>
> My legs feel lifeless. I find it difficult to even get up from the chair and walk out to the parking lot. I have to kick-start my bike, but there is no strength even to start it. The watchman helps me to kick-start the vehicle and he is surprised to see me in that state. He asks if I am alright. I say I'm fine and drive off on my bike, which is also bought on loan. I feel like a lost warrior.
>
> When I reach home, my wife is shocked to see me. After listening to what had happened in the office, she assures me that we will be fine and that I can always find another job. I feel she is much stronger than I am; she is my best support system. For the next three months, I keep applying for various posts but don't manage to pass the interviews and get a job. All my savings are over, and the EMI is due. I have no money left to even pay for the house rent.
>
> My wife suggests that we go and stay with my father, who lives with my younger brother, but I'm very hesitant to do so. However, I listen to her advice as we have no other option left. Upon arriving at my father's house, I can sense coldness from my brother. I try to be amicable, but deep down I feel suffocated.

I gently prompted Anand to dig into his subconscious for the reason behind his feeling of suffocation and discomfort with his brother. Anand immediately recollected an older memory from his present life.

> Anand: I am twenty-seven years old. My father has retired, and with his retirement money, he wants to buy a flat in my name. So he asked me to come over. I am preparing to leave when my brother calls me saying there was no need to go because father had decided to buy the flat in his (my brother's) name.
>
> I feel betrayed. I know my brother has manipulated my father. I feel very angry, but I decide to keep quiet and never ask my father again why he did what he did. I tell myself that I don't need anything; I don't need my share of my father's wealth or property, and that I shall build my own house.

I wondered at the similarity between this part of Anand's life with his past life as the zamindar in South India.

> Anand: Three days later, while I am sitting on the sofa in the living room, my younger brother rushes towards me in anger and accuses me of taking his debit card and stealing Rs 20,000. I have no clue what he is talking about and I tell him I didn't take the card. But he doesn't stop his accusations and continues to call me a thief. I am very angry and, at the same time, I also feel helpless and betrayed by my own family. I feel as if a dagger has been thrust in my heart.

This feeling of a dagger being thrust in his heart was exactly what he had experienced in his lifetime as the zamindar.

> Anand: I feel lifeless. This is the last thing I expected from my brother. I had helped him so much in his younger days, taking care of him and protecting him. And he is now calling me a thief!

Anand paused, as tears roll down his cheeks.

> Anand: Even as my brother continues his accusations, our father comes and intervenes. He tells my brother that he had taken the debit card to withdraw money to pay for expenses. I see my brother going pale for a moment, and without even saying sorry

or expressing any regret, he just walks away not realising how deeply hurt I am. I feel like a beggar. I feel like running away. I feel my legs are very weak. I feel so dependent and stuck. Although I am the eldest son, I feel I am the least important in the house.

At the end of the session, as I slowly brought my client out of his trance, I saw huge relief on his face. Anand opened his eyes: they were filled with tears. Holding my hands, he thanked me from the deepest core of his heart. He said everything in his life made sense to him now. He seemed to clearly understand the connection between his lives and the patterns flowing through them. He understood the bigger picture of his *karma* with his brother and expressed the need to let go and move on. He was clear: he did not want to die like a beggar even in this life. His joy and lightness were quite palpable.

I saw him after a week. He was jubilant! He said his legs felt strong and the pain had reduced almost by 80 per cent from what it had been earlier. He was able to walk long distances, though it would still take a while to start running. He mentioned that he felt as if the life in his legs was back. Not only that, his backache, neck pain, numbness in the hands, and the general body pain and tiredness—all had completely vanished.

The best news was that he could get back to work and had started travelling to office. In addition to all the positive physical developments, Anand said he had become a calmer person. He had calmed down and did not push his colleagues at work anymore. His peers and colleagues seemed to notice these changes in him and conveyed that he seemed like an altogether different person now!

Immediately after the first session, Anand had expressed his intense desire to walk without crutches, but he still couldn't. However, after his second session two weeks later, he was able to do so and felt great. Six weeks later, he was running down the stairs of my clinic with tears in his eyes, saying, 'I have my legs back!'

To witness such life-changing cases is the biggest reward I have gained over the course of my practice. They serve as a boost to continue with the therapy in spite of the fact that I sometimes find it painful to go through the pain of others, which surfaces during the sessions. Anand's crutch still lies with me in my clinic as a gentle reminder of this fact.

——

Naina was thirty-eight years old, employed and from a middle-class family. She was diagnosed with Systemic Lupus Erythematosus (SLE). She came to me complaining of general body and joint pains throughout the day with severe lethargy for over a year. Her medical reports indicated elevated inflammatory markers, anaemia and positive autoimmune antibodies.

Naina's regression revealed a past life in which she was a simple, middle-class woman residing in northern India at the beginning of the 20th century—a time when society was mostly male-dominated. Ill-treatment of women, even after marriage, was quite rampant across the country. In that life, Naina's relationship with her domineering husband and in-laws was further marred with suspicions on her fidelity. Eventually, the suspicion grew like a poisonous tree until, with utter hostility, they beat her to death. As Naina died in that life, the thought that impinged and penetrated deep into her consciousness was one of disbelief at being completely let down: 'My husband and his parents were supposed to protect me, but they beat me to death.'

Under normal conditions, the body's immune system protects and acts as a defense mechanism against foreign insults. But in an autoimmune disease such as SLE, the immune system turns against one's own body. It mistakenly identifies healthy tissues as foreign and vigorously attacks these cells and tissues, resulting in symptoms such as fever, malaise, joint pains, myalgia, fatigue and even temporary loss of cognitive abilities.

Through Naina's regression, I understood how this incident of the past was a metaphor in her present life. Even in the present life, her husband doubted her fidelity and was used to physically abusing her. Naina again had a strong feeling of being violated: *the person who was supposed to protect her was causing her harm.* This subconscious feeling of being let down by the one who was meant to protect her was manifesting in an exactly similar physical condition: her body's defense mechanism was attacking her tissues, joints and muscles.

I led Naina through catharsis and integration after her session. She returned after six months with normal blood count and negative autoimmune antibodies.

Interestingly, when she came for a review after eight weeks, she had eczema. Since the presentation of her skin condition was totally disconnected with her SLE, as was revealed through another regression, I present it below as a separate case to facilitate easy study and research.

—-—

Naina had severe itching resulting in violaceous patches on her legs and palms, which was not the case when I saw her the first time. When I wondered aloud if I had missed these earlier, she confirmed that they had manifested only over the past two months. While I was tempted to diagnose these rashes as a manifestation of her SLE—even though all the primary markers of SLE were receding—I did not want to be too rigid in my diagnosis. So, with an open mind, I decided to be neutral and questioned her about the development of this skin disorder.

Naina said that she felt burdened and stuck at her workplace: she deeply resented her office colleagues. She said that instead of helping her out with her heavy workload, her colleagues were *pricking* her. I found the word 'pricking' very intriguing and had an intuition that it may be the bridge that connected to the past from where this feeling originated. So, I intensified this itching feeling in Naina when she was in a state of trance. As she experienced the pricking feeling, she saw herself as an eighteen-year-old girl working in a paddy field in a village. While working, she accidentally touched a thorny bush that caused her hands and legs to bleed, and her skin turned blue.

As Naina was narrating this, she began to scratch her thighs and legs vigorously while lying in a trance in my clinic and, interestingly, the specific spot started turning blue too! From her deep subconscious state, she reported people—also workers in the paddy field—who were mere onlookers to her plight instead of helping her out of her painful situation. As Naina relived this experience of being abandoned, she also described the thorns' poisonous nature that had pricked her. I instantly realised why the locals stay away rather than approaching her: if they accidentally got pricked by the thorns in the process, they would be poisoned too. I wondered which thorn Naina was referring to, for I hadn't come across such a deadly variety during my inquisitive days at playing detective or even at the time of my rather serious study and experience in the medical field!

A quick search on Google (while she was still in a trance) revealed the existence of a specific fungus growing on sugarcane plants that rests upon the thorns, which in turn injects a natural anticoagulant, Dicumarol, from the fungus and causes bleeding in cattle when they prick them. It is nature's way of keeping cattle at bay from the nutritious and delicious sugarcane! I had come full circle in my understanding, while Naina continued to experience that life when nobody came to her rescue and she died of profuse bleeding, feeling intensely angry and helpless.

The metaphor was now quite clear to me. In her present life, Naina felt a total lack of support from her colleagues at work (rather they would criticise and humiliate her), which triggered the memory of her past life where she had been forsaken by the other workers in the field. As this memory was triggered in her subconscious in the present, the experience of being pricked by the thorns in the past surfaced. This reflected in the form of Naina's 'pricking' colleagues in her current job.

At the time of integration, I felt that the best way to enable catharsis was to guide Naina to 'remove' these thorns, one by one. It is important to note here that in regression, we begin with the premise that *reality cannot be changed—none of the events or experiences of the past can be changed—but through a psychophysical approach, the consequences of those experiences can be altered.* So, as Naina removed the thorns of her past, I assisted her in disconnecting herself from that memory which was reflecting in the form of her 'pricking' colleagues in the present.

I met Naina for a follow-up after a week. The rashes that had been so debilitating had completely disappeared, with no traces of any scars or violet patches.

With the incidence of eczema on the rise, even in younger children, this case study raises an important question: can regression help all those who are suffering from the ailment? Through my experience, I recommend that those who suffer from chronic eczema that disturbs their normal, everyday life and are dependent on medicines to suppress skin inflammation would benefit by reaching the root of this chronic condition.

——

The case of Akshara was one of my first ten in the field of regression, and it completely changed my perception of the therapy. At that time, I firmly believed that regression could treat only psychological diseases, with its scope extending to curing general body pain and minor physical disorders.

At nineteen, Akshara had been diagnosed with aplastic anaemia—a serious disorder that required her to receive blood transfusion once every three weeks. Later, as tests revealed that her bone marrow had stopped producing red blood cells, the diagnosis changed and stated the condition as Pure Red Cell Aplasia (PRCA)—a type of anaemia that affects the precursors to red blood cells but not to white blood cells. It was a very well established disorder, and as my rational mind did not foresee any scope of recovery, I was quite petrified at the idea of taking up her case for regression. But my young client talked me into it saying that she would not blame me if she did not recover and would like to give it a try all the same. I was in for the challenge.

Through regression, Akshara landed back in 1910 A.D. in central India, a time when the feudal system was largely prevalent in society. In that lifetime, she was married at a very young age and had a son. Subsequently, her husband passed away, and her life now was solely centred around her only son, who had unfortunately taken to drinking and gambling. At seventy, when the widow wanted to transfer all her property to a trust, her son demanded that she sign the papers in his name. However, she refused to do so, and in a fit of rage, he banged her head with a flower vase. The blow was fatal and she died on the spot.

I had started the session with the notion that my client must have lost a lot of blood in the past, which was reflecting in her present life, where she required a regular blood transfusion. But I was mystified with her recollection that she did not lose a drop of blood at the time of death in her past life. I was quite disappointed with this bit of information as it made no sense to me. I was just beginning to consider giving up the practice of this therapy when I had a moment of intuition: *the widow's only son, who meant everything to her and was meant to protect her, had turned against her!*

I correlated the metaphor to the molecular level, which was manifesting as such a grave disorder in Akshara's present life. Moreover, Akshara had mentioned that her uncle, who had brought her up in this life in the absence of her father, had sent her out of the house when he got married. As I could clearly see the same pattern, the same situation, the same metaphor, I was able to begin her integration by way of catharsis.

After three months, Akshara reported that her requirement for blood transfusion had gone down from once every three weeks to once every three months. Since I was still quite naive regarding the nuances of regression, I was unable to reassure her of a total recovery and lost touch with her for quite a while. At the end of almost two years, I was encouraged by the news that a surprise phone call brought me. From the other end of the line, Akshara reported that she had not required blood transfusion in the last six months and that she had started leading an everyday life.

This case was revolutionary in my practice of the therapy, for it opened my vision to some of its deeper facets. The greatest understanding, I gained from the experience is that a therapist should be willing to be open and be neutral to the facts presented through the history of the client, avoid preconceived notions, and probe deep in order to get the optimal results out of this mode of treatment.

—-—

The one theme underlying the cause of quite a few diseases that I have handled so far is fascinating: our own immune system, which is supposed to protect us, turns against our body. The emotional betrayal could come from any individual who is supposed to be a prominent part of our support system—husband, wife, mother-in-law, father—it could be anyone on whom we place our implicit trust, even a friend and not only a blood relative. A single thought carries the potential to manifest powerfully and affect the cells of our body. So metaphorically speaking, the cells that constitute my body's protection, my immune system, are targeted and affected.

Having concluded thus, I feel it necessary to clarify and explain beyond what is so apparent. I have had cases of people who have been raised in a family where all the siblings are exposed to severe hurt and betrayal by one or both of their own parents—their primary source of security. However, it is only in one particular sibling that the trauma manifests as symptoms of an autoimmune disease, while another child develops a mental disorder, and yet another remains completely sane and healthy. So that is where the need for the presence of a deep-seated memory of the past, which acts as a trigger, comes into the picture.

I can never get tired of asserting that every individual is unique; we cannot generalise. How a person reacts to a particular situation or a particular environment is based on their past: the impressions of past memories in seed-form that they carry through time. These seeds will germinate at the appropriate time when a suitable environment or situation presents itself. So, there is a vital thread that runs between the trigger, the metaphor and the seed. You may have gone through an incident of terrible betrayal in your life, where your protector or symbol of security let you down badly and went against you, but if you are not carrying the seed within from a distant past, then it is not going to manifest in you as a disease or a disorder in your present life.

Moreover, what kind of negative emotion this manifests as, depends upon the seed-memory that you carry. You have different kinds of white blood cells, like lymphocytes and neutrophils, and different kinds of memory cells. Which of these cells, tissues or parts of your body get affected is a deeper pathology, which mostly only medical professionals may understand if I try to explain. But just to satisfy the general reader's curiosity, here is an example.

Once a lady came to me with acute rheumatoid arthritis. Her regression revealed a past life where she was fatally hit on her muscles and joints by her husband. As she died in that life, she retained a strong memory: 'My muscles are hurt and my joints are broken because of my own husband.' So basically, she had invited the metaphor that 'My protection harmed me.' And the cells that provide immediate protection to these parts of the body are the neutrophils. As a result, in the present life when there was a similar situation that triggered this memory, my client developed rheumatoid arthritis, wherein her body started producing antibodies that turned against her own muscles and joints.

So, the physical memory from the past associated with that metaphor, and the emotion which constitutes the seed, is what ultimately manifests as a disease in our present life. Through regression, the person is able to integrate these three elements and arrive at an understanding, thus uprooting the seed itself and allowing wisdom to flow in its place.

Where Does the War End?
A Perspective on Chronic Conditions

Why me? How often have we asked this question as a reaction to the challenges that life throws at us? Whenever we go through a trying situation on the physical, mental, financial or any other level, we feel we are the victims of great injustice. *Why is this happening to me? What did I do to deserve this in my life?*

I discovered over time through different cases that the answer lies in these very questions.

I have had patients coming to me with headaches and body pain from which they have been suffering for a long time without any apparent cause. Both they and their doctors have failed to find any concrete answers. A classic case is that of a gentleman who had migraine. Through regression, we discovered that he had died fighting a terrible war. Imagine his situation: He is fighting a war under the bright sun. It is the most stressful time of his life. Like any warrior, the prime thought in his mind is that he must win, no matter what. For this, he must perform. It should be the best performance of his life. He is gearing himself up for striking at his foe. Suddenly, he gets hit on his head. He collapses and dies.

So, in this lifetime, whenever he is exposed to bright sunlight, or when he is stressed with the challenge to perform, he gets a migraine attack. How can you avoid the sun in daily life? And in today's world, how can you avoid stress when performance is what decides your job or whatever you do in life?

That explains how wars go beyond lives. The terrible effects of the wars of the Middle Ages or those of the Vikings and other battles, big and small, continue to trouble our minds even today, as their memories are submerged in our psyches. We aren't done with them yet. They continue to ravage us from within, in the form of cellular memories, manifesting and affecting us individually.

—–—

William, an elderly gentleman, aged about sixty, came to me with various issues. A few years before he approached me, he had been obese beyond norms, weighing a solid 400 pounds. Through external interventions and medical surgeries, he had managed to bring down his weight to 272 pounds, which was still on the higher side. His obesity had led to diabetes and hypertension. He was also suffering from a serious sleep disorder called obstructive sleep apnea—a condition in which breathing repeatedly stops and starts during sleep.

As part of our first session, I had a long conversation with him to understand where he was coming from, and about his eating habits and his lifestyle in general. His case history had interesting aspects, especially his approach and attitude to food. Below is a transcript of our conversation.

> Me: What stops you from sticking to your diet? Why don't you eat on time?
>
> William: I never know when I'm going to be full. Sometimes, I feel full early, so I stop eating; and then I feel hungry an hour later, so I eat, and that is a crazy cycle.
>
> Me: Were you obese since childhood, or did you put on weight later?
>
> William: I've been obese since childhood. When I was in sixth grade, two of my friends broke into the school office and read my health records, and we found that I was obese even when I was in kindergarten and after kindergarten, from the time I was six years

old. My father was heavy, not obese. Mother was thin.

Me: Okay. So, what do you think is the reason for your obesity?

William: I think it is biological. I've been successful in many things, but this has been a struggle forever, and I'm trying to control and manage the eating.

Me: You mean the reason for your obesity is overeating?

William: Yes....

Me: And you say you have no control over your eating; that your hand automatically reaches out for food to eat?

William: Right.

Me: And you have tried a lot of things but nothing has helped you so far?

William: Correct. Well, for short periods, I have been on an eating disorder programme with a well-known institute, and I've got some skills in maintaining my weight, but I'm not losing weight any more now. I've been eating a lot more protein; I can abstain from eating for periods of time and am able to exercise, and I've been stable. Right now, I'm at 272 pounds, and I probably would like to get down to 240.

Me: Why do you think your sugar fluctuates?

William: It's because I eat a lot of carbs. Last year, I hired a cook—and when I eat her food, I'm fine. She cooks four main meals for me.

Me: Do you cheat?

William: Yes, that's the problem. Sometimes, I'm fine and go a week or two without cheating. Then there are times when I cheat every day.

Me: When does this craving come in, making you lose control?

William: Breakdown usually happens early in the morning, when I start thinking of something I want. If I do not pay attention, it just shows up later in the day. The cravings are in my head, but I probably feel them in my chest.

Me: So, when you're gobbling, do you feel like you are filling up something that is not yours?

William: I never get full....

Me: Absolutely. I never get full.

William: Sometimes, I just don't care, and I'm eating junk.

Me: I don't care ... I eat junk ... Can you talk more on that?

William: My cook helped me throw out all the junk in my house about two or three months ago. At least for a while, even though I had cravings, I would just go on an exercise machine or read or do something. But now slowly, things have crept back in. I don't even hide them, I put them in plain sight, like I have ice cream in the freezer right now. I have some candy in the cupboard somewhere, to which I do not pay attention most of the time, but when the craving is there, I know where it is.

Other than his eating habits, the fact that he was suffering from obesity since childhood, in spite of his parents not being obese, was quite intriguing. I probed deeper and checked on the quality of his relationship with his parents. While his relationship with his mother had been quite satisfactory, the memories he had of his father were quite traumatic.

William: My father died when I was about ten years old. I was in school when it happened, and my brother found him. I was devastated, though I did not like the man. He would beat me, and I was very frightened of him, but I made my peace with him. He was trying the best he could, and when he died, I was devastated. I felt terrified and vulnerable, because I did not know who would take care of us.

I cried a lot as a kid and he wanted me to be strong, so he would constantly be yelling at me to shut up and not cry, to stop whining. I just remember him as being very harsh: when I did something wrong, he would take out his belt on me. After his death, I got over being scared; I was relieved when he died.

Initially, I felt his problems were disconnected from each other, and so I considered each of his issues as a separate entity. But when we went through the first session, I realised all his issues were interlinked. Step by step, the session unfolded well and all his physical issues connected to a single cause or memory.

> William: I'm six years old. I'm sitting at the dining table. I'm wearing boots, husky blue jeans and my favourite blue shirt. It's a Sunday morning and I'm sitting in front of food. I refuse to eat it because the eggs are touching something. And my father has just placed his belt on the table.
>
> My mother is in the kitchen. She is wearing a dark, loose dress. I am getting around the table trying to go to the kitchen to see her, but she is hiding. She does not want to deal with this.
>
> My father is sitting across the table. He is wearing a white T-shirt, tanned pants, a black belt and socks, no shoes.
>
> I'm served scrambled eggs, toast and some strawberries. I feel angry looking at the plate, as the eggs and the strawberries are touching each other. I tell myself, 'I'm not going to eat this: nobody can make me. This is not right. This is not okay. I am not going to eat this. She knows better. She knows that, then why would she do that? No, I'm not going to eat this. I'm not, I'm not, I'm NOT going to eat this!'
>
> My father, who is sitting across the table, is very angry with me. He is puffing and leaning forward angrily, yelling, 'You are going to eat this.' And I reply, 'I'm not going to eat this.' He snarls, 'You got to do it. You will sit here until you eat this.' When I refuse, he takes his belt off and puts it on the table. I am scared.
>
> I intellectually know that I should be scared, but I'm just angry and stubborn and I don't care if he gets at me with his belt. I want to run away, but he is sitting there. I keep myself focussed on the food right in front of me, and I won't look at him. He is pissed off. He pushes the chair and walks away, shouting, 'No TV, nothing for you, until you eat what is on the plate,' and I keep looking at the food remembering how angry he is.
>
> Me: What have you decided to do?

William: I'm equally stubborn. There is no way I'm going to eat that food. I sat there until 7 o'clock at night. I remember all that happened. There was no TV; I was not allowed to do anything. I had to sit there with this fucking plate in front of me. I would not eat anything and, finally, they asked me to go to bed. I did not eat anything that day, because I was not going to eat the breakfast at all.

I am shaking right now. I will remember this for the rest of my life. I will never forget this. I will never forget this day, never.

Me: What are your feelings about your father?

William: I will not submit; I will never submit. I will not do what he wants me to do. I will not do it. I keep looking at the food over and over to keep remembering how angry I am. I will not do what he wants me to do. I will not eat this crap.

Me: How are you feeling when you watch your father taking out his belt to punish you?

William: I'm feeling scared. I'm feeling very scared. To not feel scared, I look away, I look at the food. It is my will over his.

At this juncture, I nudged William to go further back in time, to find the source of this deep fear in him that was evoked just by looking at his father's belt. And he regressed to a time when he was younger.

William: I'm five years old. I'm beaten with a belt.

I was playing outside; it was a holiday. He was sleeping because he worked nights, and I woke him up. He brought me into the house and yelled at me, and he took his belt off and beat me with it. I just kept watching him beating me without understanding why! I was very scared....

As I kept nudging William to connect with his emotions, I could sense a deep fear in him, a fear of being punished. Suddenly, from his state of trance, he began referring to the recurring dreams that he used to have when he was younger and to which he had referred even at the time of giving his history. In the dream, he saw himself entering a basement full of dead bodies, which filled him with despair and terror. I could not ignore this reference to the dream in the middle of his session. Intuitively, I felt that his fear and sense of rebellion towards his father had a much deeper root, perhaps beyond the present.

> Me: The tightness, the fear, the restlessness, feel them more and more. I am going to count you backwards from five to zero, and you will move back in time to another place, another time, another life, the source of this deep fear of being attacked, of being killed, of being punished. The dead bodies, how and why they haunt you....

William effortlessly regressed into a past life.

> William: It is a concentration camp. I'm in a wooden shack, with I think forty to fifty people. I see dead bodies when I walk. It looks like I'm in the 1940s.
> I'm a fourteen or fifteen-year-old boy. I'm wearing a dark shirt and pants, and sandals. The colour of my skin is white, but I am filthy, dirty. I need a shower. I'm smelling terrible. The smell is horrendous all over. I try not to smell. I try to breathe through my mouth because the smell is horrible. The smell of death, faeces, sweat, vomit.
> It is cold. Basically, I am numb. I'm just numb from it all, the smell, the cold, the ugliness, the horror. I know that I have gone through a lot, the horror, the terror, the fear. It is all there, but I've just numbed myself to it all. Yeah, I cannot live with all of it. I am sort of waiting to die.
> I am one of the youngest in there, and everybody is just kind of vacant-looking. I look away. It is too hard to see them. It is too hard. I cannot make out their faces. It is too hard to look at them. I do not want to connect with them. I want to be by myself. They don't have to give me anything; I cannot give them anything. We just do what we need to do. I do not talk to them much. I am sort of lost inside myself. I don't even know.... I am just lost. I go someplace else. It is like when I am meditating. I just

go someplace else. I am not present. There is nothing to run away from or to. It is like I'm just there. When I look or pay attention, it is horror. Yes ... anywhere but right here where I am. This is horrible ... horrible....

I pick up dead bodies. They give me some food that I do not like, but I eat it because my body needs something. The stuff feels like slop. It feels like oatmeal and some other stuff thrown in. I am actually not hungry; I do not care. I know I have to eat. I try not to taste the food. I take it in because I know the body needs it, but I know if I could I would not eat at all. I don't like the food: it is ugly.

Me: The food is ugly, but you eat to survive....

William: Yes.

Me: And as you are filling up your stomach, what is going on in your mind?

William: I get full quickly, and sometimes I even give food to other people because I do not eat all that they give me. I do not like it. I just eat what I think I need to eat so I can keep going.

They serve the food in a metal plate, which has divisions, like a military plate. But the food is always just the same: they serve just a ladle of the stuff. And I do not think they even give me a fork. I think I use my fingers to eat.

There is no humanity there. You just live to kind of take care of yourself. It is not like the stories that I remember hearing about concentration camps, (connecting from current life) but it is worse than that, for me at least.

Me: Such a terrible place ... After eating the food, where are you going?

William: They line me up. I am in a line and I take bodies out of this dark basement and put them on a cart and take them some place. Sometimes, I just drop them in a pile or sometimes ... terrible ... terrible. There is excrement, there is ... terrible ... And I usually get to hold the bodies' feet. They have all died in a gas chamber. I puke. I am crying. I too am going to be there one day. That's *me* in the future.

The memory of the horror of that particular life, which William had regressed to, had been so deeply embedded in him that his body started reacting in the present even as he recounted the events from his past. He was nauseous and said that he felt like vomiting.

> Me: You are living in constant fear that your fate is going to be like that one day....
>
> William: My chest is tight. I am living in constant fear of death. I am numb. I know something bad will happen, but there is a place inside me that does not care what they do to me. I mean, I don't care what they do to me.
>
> Me: Feel that rebel inside you rising ... Feel that stubbornness ... You don't care what they do to you....
>
> William: Yes, they have taken everything. I don't have anything. They can't hurt me anymore.
>
> Me: Can't hurt me anymore ... They have taken everything from me....
> As I count from five down to zero, you will move back in time, the time when you were still free and not in the camp, the time when you were happy and with your family and free.

With this, William regressed further in time.

> William: I can see the house. It's a wooden house, and there are nice trees in the neighbourhood. It is busy, with carts and cars and climbers on the street. The wooden house where we live is colourful. The ceiling is coated with stucco, a light fixture though. There is a hallway inside with stairs. It's not a big house. There is a language being spoken, which I don't understand. I assume it is German. I am a kid, and I don't understand what they are saying. I am a little overweight, chubby. The colour of my skin is white and I have red hair.
> Father is a merchant; he sells things. Mother stays at home. Father is a little overweight. He doesn't smile. He is very stern. I am scared of him. He is all for fairness, in that he supports me. I

know the rules; I know what I am supposed to do. I am a good kid.

I have an older brother who works with my dad. He is out of school. I think he is seventeen, and I am thirteen. Brother takes care of me. He plays with me when he has time. Usually, I want to do more things with him when he has the time for it.

I like my mother. She makes good food. My mom and dad have their respective roles and they play them out well. There is usually not a lot of conflict. After school, I play soccer with my friends. We play around in the neighbourhood and then I go home for dinner. Everybody eats together around six o'clock. Life is easy. It is good. I enjoy myself. I am most of the time comfortable and at ease. I feel safe.

But I think I am getting concerned and worried over all the stuff being talked about. It is a Jewish home so they have talked about pilgrims in the past, and I know they are worried about it, but I am not paying attention to it.

Military comes down the street with vehicles and everybody is trying to close themselves up in their homes and shutting the doors. It is a loud noise. We go back to our daily businesses but much more tense and more anxious and concerned. People are talking about it all the time, and I just don't want to listen to it. I don't want to pay attention to that. I want to play soccer and be with my brother and my friends.

Parents are discussing about moving. My father does not want to move. My mother wants to move. There is tension. I am starting to pay attention to the fact that all is not okay. I am starting to get scared. I don't know why.

Then we were rounded up within a square. I get separated from my family. My brother and my parents go into one group, and I go into another group. I don't see them again. I am scared, sad.

People come in uniforms and they are pushing us into trucks. I am trying to lift myself into the truck and this guy pushes me hard. There is a lot of pushing. I can't see much, and we are driven off. We are taken to the train and put in it. There are a lot of people, almost no standing room. I stand for a long time until I can't stand anymore. I try to sit but there is no room to sit. Then the smell starts because there are no bathrooms, and the smell is horrendous. I am hungry because there is no food. And the hunger is very strong ... After a while, I just go numb.

I am supposed to be hungry as I have not eaten in a while. I am totally shutting down. I am just not there. I am someplace else. I can tell you everything around me. I can tell you what is going on, but I am not feeling anything. I am just not there. It is like all of us are alone in this terrible place, in this terrible situation, yet all not there.

I am on the train and I don't care where I am going, that does not matter. They take me to a camp and I get off the train. I can barely walk. They are separating us into groups. I don't know which group I am in, but they are taking my clothes off with everybody else's. My eyes are sunken and my job is to take the dead people.

I feel so forsaken. I feel so overwhelmed. I can't allow that feeling. I push it away but it keeps coming back. I keep wondering when it's going to be my turn to die. This is it. This is life. This is what it is. I know my family is dead. There is no future. There is nothing.

I just see many dead bodies being picked up. I know that my family is in the other group, while I have been in the group that stays alive. They were left in the first group to die. I have no hope of ever seeing them again. No hope of the life that we had, to return to.

Me: What is your name?

William: They call me Erik.

After I finish my shift of picking and piling the bodies, the guards come in and ask me to go with them. They put me into another dormitory with people I don't know. The next day, they tell me I have to take a shower and so take off all my clothes. They put me into the gas chamber. While there, some of us know what is going to happen, and some of us don't. A lot of people believe they are going to have a shower. The gas comes out and I breathe it in as fast as I can.

I want to breathe in as fast as I can, and I am frightened. I just want it to be over. And as I breathe it in, I start choking. I do not smell it. I feel it going into my nose, burning. My nose is very sensitive and I start choking.

Me: As you are breathing fast and taking in the gas, feel the smoke. What is the smoke doing to your chest?

William: I am hurting, choking, coughing, and I am looking forward to dying. I do not know when I died, but I know that my spirit stayed with my body. I am sort of alive inside the dead body, but my heart has stopped. My eyes are open even though I am not seeing anything. I think that this is what it is like to be dead, knowing that there would be somebody else like me who is going to pick up my body and put it in a pile … I am feeling free and am sort of waiting and open for whatever was going to happen next.

William's regression had taken him back to the time when he had lived as a happy Jewish boy and later had been sent to a Nazi concentration camp. This was the time around the Second World War. He had died choking in a gas chamber, which could be linked with his chronic asthma in his present lifetime.

As he spent meaningless days in the concentration camp, there was a feeling of intense rebellion inside him because of the way they were treated under the Nazi regime. He was deprived of proper food, and he carried that traumatic memory with him even when he died in that lifetime. In his present life, this memory was triggered when his father punished him rather harshly for something. 'You will not do what you want to do; you will only listen to me,' shouting thus, he had made the young lad sit at the dining table trying to force him to eat the food laid before him, throwing a leather belt in front of him and threatening, 'If you don't eat that, I'm going to punish you.'

I could gather from whatever William was narrating in a subconscious state that his father intended to thrash him with the belt, in case he disobeyed. After sitting at the table for twelve hours at a stretch, without eating, William rebelled: 'Damn it! I'm not going to eat what you want me to eat. I will eat *everything* that you don't want me to eat.' With this, the memory of his intense feeling of rebellion towards the way he was suppressed in the concentration camp during the Nazi regime got triggered instantly.

And from then onwards—from the age of six—he started putting on weight. He rebelled against his father and went out to eat junk food. He started eating all kinds of unhealthy food just to prove to his father that he couldn't be controlled by him. But sadly for him, and clearly to me, what young William failed to see at that tender age was that he was only hurting himself in the whole process. With this understanding coming to me, I now had the job of passing the same knowledge over to William which, I knew, would facilitate his healing journey. So, I began the process of integration.

When William initially shared his history with me, before we went through his regression, I noticed what was bothering him the most because he was unable to understand and accept why he was going through so many issues at the same time. He was frustrated at being addressed as fat and lazy by the world around him. I could see that he was fighting with himself all the time: 'Why am I not able to control my eating habits? Why am I like this? Look at me, I'm ...' He was at war with himself, feeling singled-out by life, and he did not know where the roots of his woes lay.

I could empathetically relate to his confusion and trauma: constant medication for hypertension and obesity, with side-effects; insulin injections thrice a day for diabetes; and feeling lethargic and sleepy during the day due to improper sleep at night. I mean, it was enough to drive anyone crazy! No wonder, William said that he often felt he was living like a slave, and his regression threw light on that feeling of his. We realised that the roots of his problems lay in a deep trauma created in a concentration camp, in the 1930s. That experience embedded in him the need to rebel. That rebellion didn't do him any good, but made him obese in this lifetime—and obesity is a precursor for diabetes, hypertension and upset sleep patterns. So, when William developed sleep apnea, he could not sleep well, and as a result, he would wake up feeling tired and irritated.

During the integration, I guided William to get the whole picture clear in his conscious mind, which his subconscious had so graphically revealed during the regression. He needed to understand the root cause of all his present issues—the traumatic memory of his past in the concentration camp; how it was triggered in his current life, and how each of his physical issues connected with each other. As he understood everything, he became open and willing to participate in his healing process.

When I reviewed him after a gap of time, it was a much more positive, clear and calm William that I spoke to. He said that on the very next day after his regression, he was passing by McDonald's, and he felt initially tempted to indulge his taste buds. But a voice inside him firmly said, 'No, no more. You're not going to go there.' And he obeyed the voice, without any feeling of being controlled or sense of rebellion.

As a therapist, it was rewarding to know that my client was finally beginning to hear himself. The last time I spoke to him, he revealed that he had lost twenty pounds. His BP and diabetes were now under control with medications, and although he still used the machine to cope with sleep apnea, it was sure to be resolved if he continued to lose weight at the same pace. The intensity of his asthma attacks and medication had also reduced.

— — —

Irritable Bowel Syndrome, or IBS, is a very common condition. At least one in ten people suffer from this disorder at some point in their lives. One of the primary causes of this disorder is believed to be a faulty signaling between the brain and gut, and its classic symptoms include bloating of the stomach, incontinence and constipation. IBS is usually diagnosed by a presentation of typical symptoms rather than medical tests, as there is no specific pathology that can establish the presence of the disease.

Asad, a thirty-four-year-old dynamic IT professional, came to me with symptoms of this disorder from which he had been suffering for the last twenty years. While he reported frequent abdominal pain and cramps and constant changes in his bowel habits and movements, his biopsy and scan reports were completely normal. At the time of taking his history, I was able to sense him reflecting fear, helplessness and embarrassment in his life's pursuits and endeavours. Sensing a connection between these emotions and his physical issues, I suggested that we go through regression.

During his regression, Asad saw himself as a twenty-five year old Greek prince who had promised his mother, the queen, that he would win his maiden war and return victorious. Although he embarked with a lot of energy and enthusiasm, he failed to plan properly for the attack, because he had received wrong information about the enemy's army movements.

On seeing the opponent's army on the battlefield, he was shaken, as he realised that his army's strength was weaker than his enemy's. Yet he fought a losing battle, because the thought of being unable to fulfil his promise brought him unimaginable shame. Ultimately, the enemy's troops surrounded him, cut open his abdomen, took out his gut and wore it as a trophy around their neck. His dying thought was, 'It is a big dishonour for a prince to die losing a battle.' Later, I searched on the Internet, and to my shock and disgust, I found that wearing a slain opponent's gut as a trophy was indeed a custom in the olden days of war!

What did Asad's past life have to do with his bowel disorder in the present? Well, through regression, we further discovered that at the age of sixteen in his current life, Asad was an intelligent boy bubbling with energy. He studied both mathematics and science in high school and excelled in both the subjects. However, in the final examination, he did not perform well and failed to live up to his teachers' expectations.

The whole episode of working hard but failing to perform successfully brought about great embarrassment and developed into an escalating fear of failure in my client. This had an impact on Asad's bowel habits, which became inconsistent and irregular. The emotions that were triggered by his failure in the examination, in turn, triggered the latent memory of his horrifying death in his past life as a Greek prince. In both the lives he was unable to live up to others' expectations of him. In both the lives, he had failed to keep up his promise successfully. In the past, he had lost his gut as a result of failure, and the same thing metaphorically repeated itself in his present life—his gut and intestines failed to function properly, even in the present, which became the cause for the development of IBS in his system. Interestingly, the disorder would trigger only when he was under stress to perform.

During integration, I guided Asad to suggest to his conscious and subconscious mind, gently, but firmly that the war of the Greek prince was over and done with. He no longer had to keep fighting—either outside or inside himself. With an assimilation of this understanding, I closed his session. Three months later, when I called him to my clinic for a review, I was happy to see that he had healed convincingly. Asad said his bowel movements had been quite normal over the past three months, which was a big surprise and quite out of the ordinary compared to what he had been undergoing in the last twenty years. Since the understanding he gained from his regression, Asad has not reported any symptoms of IBS till now.

—

Once I had to deal with a strange case of migraine where the headache was so intense that my client, Asha, also suffered from blindness in one eye. Most doctors would not believe her, but a neurologist said she had retinal migraine. She had approached me asking whether I believed her and if so, would I be able to help her? I told her that I took a neutral stance with all my clients and simply flowed with the course of healing that unfolded during regression. I also confirmed that the neurologist was right about the diagnosis.

Asha agreed and shared her concerns with me. She complained of severe migraine in the front portion of the left side of the head. The headache was usually accompanied by total blindness in the left eye. Most doctors had concluded her headache-induced blindness to be psychosomatic, which had left her feeling very frustrated.

As I probed into Asha's history, she revealed that she felt very scared and guilty about not taking care of her family. If her daughter was unwell, she would neither eat nor sleep, and if inevitably she had to leave her, she would do so only after ensuring that her husband was in her place, watching their daughter. Even then, she would quickly return and take her place by her daughter's side.

As my client narrated this, I noticed her left eye starting to flutter and water. I found this quite unusual because normally when you cry, tears flow from both eyes. But in her case, only her left eye was watering. I also noticed her absentmindedly touching the left side of her head, which gave me a clue that there was a link between her feeling scared about not being able to take care of her family and her migraine with blindness in her left eye.

Through regression, we discovered that in one of her past lives, she had been happily living as the wife of the chief priest of a temple in a popular pilgrimage centre in the state of Gujarat in West India. All was well in that lifetime, until one night, a masked man entered their house and killed the priest, her husband. He was about to kill even their five-year-old son, but the mother (Asha, in this life) came in between and the dagger pierced her left eye, blinding that eye completely. As she realised that the masked intruder was none other than her slain husband's brother, who wanted the priest's position, she begged him to let her go with her son and daughter, promising that she would never return or come in his way.

Thus Asha, in her past life, left home with her children, desolate and shelter-less, and ended up leading an impoverished life on a railway platform and eating from trash. One day she collapsed, and the onlookers thinking her to be dead, took her to the hospital. When she regained consciousness and returned to the railway platform, she was shocked to find her children missing. She wandered in search of them for many days but was unable to find them. Finally, she died, lying listlessly under a tree, feeling wretched and miserable with the thought that she had been unable to look after her children. At the time of her death, she cursed, 'God is so ruthless. Why did he give humans life if he had to make us suffer like this?'

The memory of this past life was triggered in her present life when Asha, as a fifteen-year-old girl, was taken to a leper's home on a field trip from her school. She had entered the home happily but the moment she saw the thin, emaciated woman with leprosy in a white saree, she became unconscious and had collapsed. She had woken up with a mild headache, saying to herself, 'What is this? Why did God give life if He had to make human beings suffer in this manner?' That incident triggered the memory of her dying moments in her past life as an emaciated woman separated from her children.

However, Asha was not troubled by bouts of headache until she was twenty-two-year-old, and her brother went through a divorce. She was not able to help him through it. She carried a lot of guilt because of that, which was an intensifying factor for her headache. When she got married and had a daughter, she would constantly keep an eye on her whenever she fell sick, because she felt that if she didn't do so, she would lose the chance of taking care of her family.

Basically, my client was driven by guilt and fear. That is when her migraine would be at its worst, even causing blindness in her left eye—the memory of the dagger piercing her left eye as she was trying to protect her son in her past life. Interestingly, Asha's brother in her present life was her son in her past life, and her present life daughter was her daughter in her past life, too.

After the session, everything looked fine and Asha went home feeling quite relieved. But she came back after two or three weeks saying she was suffering from headaches again. Now the pain was in the back portion of the left side of her head instead of the front. So, we decided to go through one more session to trace out the root.

During her session, Asha once again travelled back in time, to yet another lifetime, when she was a soldier who had been ordered by the king to kill a young child. The soldier's conscience pricked him at the thought of carrying out such a heinous act; he was reminded of his promise to his three-year-old son that he would come back for him. It was almost two years since he had left home to fight in terrible wars.

In the end, he refused to carry out his king's orders. The king got angry and killed the soldier by striking him hard on the back of the left side of his head with the butt of his sword. The soldier's dying thought was, 'I obeyed the king and did terrible things in my life, so I deserve to be punished.' Thus, in this lifetime, the soul assumed the form of a weak lady to wipe out the impressions from the past life of a soldier.

After this session, Asha completely recovered from her migraine. I have been following up with her for more than a year now. Her headache is totally gone and there are absolutely no symptoms of blindness in her eye.

—-—

These studies reveal how we are capable of storing, carrying and manifesting memories in the present of unpleasant incidents which have occurred many years ago in the past. Washing away memories of wars or battles, as the ones described above in the cases of my clients, is easier said than done. Though the war, or even a conflict between individuals, may have ended many centuries ago, it still goes on and is reflected not only within an individual as a physical disorder or disease, but even around them in the form of prejudices and aggressive behaviour towards others.

In another interesting case, my client belonged to a wealthy family of landlords. He was constantly engaged in a family feud. I could sense a lot of anger in him because of his inability to accept and understand the hostility between the families. In fact, he confessed that they carried so much of hatred for each other that they wouldn't even mind slitting the throats of each other or their family members.

When we explored his subconscious through regression, we discovered that in one of his previous lifetimes, he and his brother had been great friends and partners in a successful shipping business somewhere in Great Britain. But my client, out of greed, backstabbed his brother and poisoned him to death to grab the entire business and its profits in his sole name. The brother who died carried the memory of this betrayal through lifetimes, and the conflict between the two brothers in the present was a manifestation of this memory of the past.

My client confirmed that he and his brother were at war with each other right from childhood and that his brother had always been inclined to take away things that rightfully belonged to him. I was amazed at the revelations, and even more at what happened thereafter.

As my client developed complete clarity of the past and present through his session, he was filled with wisdom and understanding about his seemingly never-ending war with this brother. He was able to accept the situation wholeheartedly, and his mind calmed down. He reported that three days later, after his session, he had been to meet his brother and, with tears in his eyes, had explained everything to him. On hearing the whole story, his brother melted and hugged him, saying, 'Let's end it. We've fought enough.'

Thus, a war-like situation in a family, which could have led to the death of people, was resolved through a 360-degree understanding of the situation—why it is the way it is and accepting it the way it is.

—-—

Wars have a much more devastating and lasting impact than the rational mind can ever think of or imagine. Though the fight may have ended a century or two ago, memories are embedded in the subtle body, which in turn manifest as physical problems in a lifetime even after a thousand or two thousand years since it actually happened. These manifestations may include chronic conditions like migraine, obesity, hypertension, sleep disorders, general body pain, a deep phobia and so on, in the individual who carries memories of the war he was a part of. Take, for example, the Nazi regime during the Second World War. The condition of the people who lived in the concentration camps was so terrible that they carry deep traumas, which affect them through lifetimes and which come to light during sessions with clients.

So, where does the war truly end? My guide in worldly and spiritual matters used to say, 'The only thing I can change in this world is myself. When *I* change, the whole world changes with me.' Through my professional and personal life, I have grown to embrace this pearl of wisdom. The biggest war lies within us, and most of our sufferings are a result of this conflict within us. We have fought wars—both gory and petty—many years or lifetimes ago, without being aware that their effects can travel beyond real-time. Can we totally nullify the effects? In my experience, it depends on each one of us. We may choose to carry the hurt and trauma into further lifetimes, or we may decide to make peace with the situation simply by accepting it—as life is presented to us in the form of trials and challenges.

Each lifetime is but a culmination of many previous lives. It is not my intention at all to intimidate you with the idea of *karma* or the proverbial 'as you sow, so shall you reap principle'. If there is anything that has deeply touched my being during sessions with my clients, it is the knowledge and understanding that the suffering of people is real. And the one who makes light or humour of it is none but a sadist.

What I want to share is what I have observed and learnt as the way *through* these sufferings, if not *out* of them. To my understanding, that is just one: the way of acceptance.

We Are Not Only Our Genes
The Role of Epigenetics in Causing Health Disorders, Obesity, Diabetes and Hypertension

What came first: the chicken or the egg? I have always been intrigued by this million-dollar age-old question. How I wish I knew the answer! Probing into the cause of chronic diseases, I now raise a question that may invite a similar debate: *Are we defined by our genes, or do we define our genes?*

To say that obesity runs in the family is partly right because when the parents are obese or overweight, it is likely that the weight of the newborn child is also more than the usual norm. There may also be a situation where the newborn baby weighs normal, but as she grows up, she may be in an environment where there is a casual attitude towards eating. Discipline in food habits may be lacking, and the child may grow up with the tendency to eat unhealthy food just like her parents. In retrospect, are the genes causing the child to be obese or is the child choosing to be born in a womb with genes such that she grows up to be obese?

The term 'retro-diagnosis' has been popping up in my mind since the past few years. Simply put, it refers to a diagnosis based on the imitation of the style or pattern from the past into the present. In some very interesting cases during regression, I found that clients with obesity generally had a past life where they died as a beggar or as a homeless person, hungry, thirsty and emaciated. So, in the next lifetime, they chose a womb where they were sure to find enough blubber to survive. I have come across cases of fibromyalgia as a manifesting condition of the body when it remembers the pain and physical trauma that it underwent from abuse and torture during the World Wars.

A common cause of eczema is living and dying in severe cold in the past, with nothing to cover the body or parts of the body. As a result, when there is a similar situation causing the skin to be exposed and dry up in the current life, the memory of that lifetime is triggered and the body manifests it in the form of eczema.

In some people, the rate of metabolism is better, that is, they burn calories faster than others. Well, that's of course because of the genes. But the moot question here is: *why did I choose to be born with that particular set of genes?* This can be answered only when we allow our minds to open up to the idea of existence beyond the physical, for such choices are purely made by the soul in its journey of evolution. Of course, chronic health conditions are genetic, but they are also 'Para genetic'—something that goes beyond genes and anything physical. Such a choice happens at the soul-level; it is the soul's plan to be delivered out of such a womb. Sometimes, it is sucked into a new womb as soon as it leaves the old body, to process its evolutionary plan. In short, I *choose* to have certain physical features and for that, I need a particular set of genes, so I am born out of a womb that can provide me with the suitable DNA.

In a family, children tend to take over one parent's features in a dominant way: 'Why am I not more like my mother? Why do I look like my father? Look at my dark skin …' and there's a big fight between the siblings. Is this really genetics? In his groundbreaking research, Dr Michael Newton follows the choices that souls make between lives and why we choose certain bodies to reincarnate. Regression cannot change *our* choice of physical attributes, whether ugly or beautiful, fair or dark, short or tall. Still, it helps us become aware and conscious so that acceptance of our present condition becomes easy and simple.

In the light of the evidence collected during the course of therapy with my clients, I conclude that such chronic health conditions are not purely genetic, because, basically, we are choosing our genes and subsequently the womb which carries those genes. The question here is, while we choose to be born in a particular way, do we need to continue to remain as we are born? That's where conditioning, or what Bruce Lipton in his book *The Biology of Belief* refers to as 'epigenetics', comes into the picture. The environment around the genes can affect the genes and actually change the composition of the DNA. Coming back to the question on genes that I posed at the start of this chapter, I make bold to assert that we *can* define our genes to a significant extent and subsequently who we are and what we become.

—-—

A forty-year old man came to me complaining of chronic acidity and obesity. He said both his parents suffered from the same health condition, so initially, we were tempted to conclude it as a genetic condition. However, through regression, we discovered that as a seven year old boy, he had gone through a very stressful episode related to his father's financial crunch. His father had lost his job and was under heavy debt, which he was unable to repay and so was constantly trying to dodge money-lenders. One night, the lenders barged into his house and woke up his sleeping son—my client—threatening him with dire consequences if he did not reveal the whereabouts of his father. The tender boy was tongue-tied with fear and confusion, until his mother came and handled the situation. After that, he was prone to sleeplessness and nightmares, and consequently, he developed acidity. On probing further, it was also revealed that his mother developed acidity only after her husband had lost his job, and her husband developed the same condition after he incurred a loss in his business! Strangely, my client confided that his siblings did not suffer from acidity.

My conclusion is that he was genetically predisposed to acidity, which, in turn, made him susceptible to environmental factors. Thus, both genetics *and* epigenetics contributed to his acidity. We also found out that the emotion of insecurity backed his obesity. On many days, he had to go without food or just with one meal a day due to his family's poor financial condition during his childhood. As a result, he started eating uncontrollably whenever he could lay hands on food. Even as he grew up and became financially successful, his tendency to gorge continued, making him obese. Now, he was not genetically predisposed to obesity—neither of his parents were obese. This was purely epigenetics at play. The gentleman lost five kilograms within three months from his regression sessions, and he was off his acidity medication soon after. He has also been completely cured of insomnia and recurring nightmares.

So, our genetic make-up, for sure, is a base that predisposes individuals to certain health conditions. For example, fair-skinned people are more susceptible to cancer when they are exposed to sun rays. Children born of obese parents are generally predisposed to developing obesity. But at the same time, the environment is also important.

Now the hypothesis that we are able to modify the environment around our genes means we are capable of changing our destiny, but we cannot change the physical part of it. A person cannot turn fair from being dark, or grow tall from being very short—no, the physical aspect remains the same. Then how does the change manifest? By understanding how mental conditioning works and affects our overall health, we can in turn, perceive the play of epigenetics, and work out ways to make the desired changes.

--

Chronic diseases mostly have their roots in our childhood. If they are uprooted as they set in, much of our turmoil later can be avoided. But once the roots are embedded deeply, it is not only difficult to uproot but even tough to contain the resulting weed that is likely to grow out of proportion. Similarly, the little oaths or pledges that we make in our childhood knowingly or unknowingly add on as time passes, and cause more harm to the self than one can imagine. We often make little oaths, out of ignorance, in our daily lives. For example, in the event of a fight with my best friend, I am likely to swear in anger: 'I will never come to your house again.' But after a week when I realise I can't stay without him, I end up being generous—more with myself than with my friend—and tell myself, 'It's okay; I can go.' We are back to being best friends again and all is well.

I took an oath that I will never enter my friend's house again because of how he behaved, but my will was not strong enough to back it up. In other words, the feeling of love or forgiveness is stronger, which makes us let go of what we had decided earlier. Our ability to forget the incident takes over and helps us to make a fresh beginning. When the art of forgetting and forgiving with love comes into play, the pledge or oath that we might have made some time ago is overruled. It dissolves in the warmth of these rather divine qualities.

Now imagine another situation where our little oath is backed by a powerful will and a strong negative emotion, which is usually anger, guilt, sadness or deep regret. What happens? The oath remains little no longer, but it takes on a huge proportion—just like the little weed that grows out of size if it isn't uprooted in its early stages. It impacts our health by conditioning our mind to think in the direction of fulfilment of our oath, or in other words, creating a set pattern of our thinking. These patterns of thoughts are what constitute the environment around our genes, which Lipton refers to as epigenetics in his book, and which in esoteric or spiritual terms is known as the 'subtle body'.

When we take a powerful oath out of great anger or profound sadness, the charge carried by these negative emotions gets stored in our body in the form of cellular memory. Each time we think of the oath, or say or do something related to it, we are storing additional negative energy in our body. Drop by drop, we are allowing the empty bucket to be filled up to the brim until it can hold no more, and the water finally overflows. The manifestation of chronic health conditions, such as diabetes, hypertension, obesity, asthma, and even cancer are a result of such an overflow of negative charge in our body, which has been accumulating bit by bit over a period of time. Every little thought, word or deed in the direction of the fulfilment of the oath counts. The negative energy stored in our cells remodels the body tissues and manifests as chronic diseases. Evidently, healing from such diseases occurs when we break the thinking pattern that has set in and release ourselves from these self-created mental bindings.

My finding is that the effect of such strong mental-conditioning can last through lifetimes, especially if an oath is taken at the time of death. For example, once a gentleman came to me to cure his squint and over his history, I could make out that he had a strange fear of getting married and having a family. He was already sixty when I saw him. His regression revealed a lifetime when he was a Red Indian who had been pierced in one eye by the enemy's arrow. His tribe and village had been plundered by a neighbouring tribe, and his entire family consisting of his wife and children were killed when he was out hunting. He was filled with deep anguish that he had been unable to protect and save his family. Subsequently, he succumbed to the wound in his eye, and at the time of his death, he took an oath that he would never again raise a family, because the loss brings unbearable pain and the guilt of not being able to protect them.

I am sure he would have reconsidered making such a strong mental decision if only he had known that it would keep him company through several lifetimes!

Another time, a young man of twenty-five came to me complaining of chronic stomach pain—cramps that were stabbing in nature. As I gained his trust, he confided that he was also gay.

He said he found women very vulnerable and weak—and I found that quite a strange reason for his sexual aversion to women. His sessions revealed that he had been a strong soldier in one of his past lives, whose wife and daughter were raped and killed by his own friends in his absence.

He had left home saying he was going for some work, but the fact was that he was seeing other women and had gone out to have fun with them. His lusty friends knew about his true whereabouts and they had taken advantage of his absence from home. As the soldier returned home and discovered what had happened, he was filled with inconsolable remorse and stabbed himself in his stomach with his sword. He was filled with terrible guilt that his thirst for carnal pleasure had cost him the lives of his wife and daughter. He died with a strong thought: 'My desire for women took away everything from me; I shall never look at a woman again.'

In the current life, as he reached puberty and his hormones started playing their role, the oath of his past life surfaced. Who else could he turn to for his sexual needs, if not women? Obviously, it had to be another man.

There was more to this case, because the past is, after all, just a skeleton. What provides flesh and blood to the skeleton and gives it shape and life is the current life. That is why, from the perspective of regression therapy, our present life is as relevant as past lives, and that is where mental conditioning comes into the picture. In the case of the gay man, he had secretly witnessed his uncle forcing himself upon his mother in his father's absence in childhood. He had pretended to be asleep, but was internally seething with anger and helplessness that he had been unable to protect his mother.

He felt guilty, and at the same time, developed a strong feeling that having sex with a woman was terrible and amounted to hurting her. At that moment, he concluded that he would never hurt a woman, and because he associated sex with hurt, his subconscious decided never to have sex with a woman. As he reached puberty, he would look at women but would never feel attracted to them—a manifestation of his oath from his past life, triggered in his current life.

I will return to this subject later and touch upon the sensitive aspects of parental and mass conditioning. Still, for the moment, this prelude should be sufficient to provide an insight into the cases that are going to be discussed ahead.

--

Diabetes and hypertension are pandemic health conditions, the causes of which doctors and therapists mostly trace to unhealthy lifestyles. When I initially started treating clients for these diseases through regression, I believed their source to be some deep-rooted problem from the past. However, as I progressed with my practice, I realised that the root cause of these diseases did not lie in the past as much as it did in the mind—in the way we think, or how our mind is conditioned to think. Basically, these are not *only* lifestyle diseases, but are also, what I would term as 'mindset diseases'. If my mindset is right, I will not choose an unhealthy lifestyle.

A gentleman in his late forties came to me with an issue of uncontrolled diabetes. He was the CEO of a very big company and materially he had nothing to complain about. But for quite some time, he had been struggling to keep his sugar-level under control, and also mildly suffered from hypertension and lack of sleep. During our first meeting, I found him to be very fidgety and restless, which evoked my curiosity to explore the source of his restlessness. As my client relaxed and gently slipped into the subconscious state, his mind took him back to a time in his current life when he was about twelve years old. From his subconscious state, he revealed that as a child, he belonged to a middle-class family. His father was under the heavy burden of loans and was constantly struggling to meet his son's needs.

'I'm studying and my spectacles break,' whispered my client. 'The pair has already broken twice, but I am still using it by tying and repairing it with a thread. Finally, it has given up. I go and tell my father, 'Look, I need a new pair of spectacles now. Enough is enough.' But all that my father says is, 'Sorry, I can't afford to buy you a new pair now. Please repair it again and use the same pair.' My client stated that he was very upset when he heard this from his father. He also saw himself crying inconsolably and at the same time thinking about what to do in the situation. In the end, he concluded vehemently, 'I'm not going to stretch my hands in front of my father anymore. I shall make my own money. I shall stand up for myself so that I don't have to beg from anybody.'

Now that decision was so powerfully willed that his life changed afterwards. From an average student, he turned into a very bright student and he started topping his class. He went on to get a distinction in his tenth grade, joined IIT, then IIM, and had a very successful career. At forty-five, he had totally forgotten the little incident with his father that had actually triggered him to toil with a vengeance, and, while thirty long years had passed since he took his oath, it was still driving all his endeavours.

The fire that he had lit long ago was still ablaze. He wasn't eating and sleeping on time, and as stress built up in his body, his pancreas stopped functioning optimally leading to diabetes. Due to chronic stress and pressure, his tissues started remodelling, his arteries became stiff and, finally, he also developed hypertension.

In another instance, a hardworking thirty-six-year-old IT professional came in with a clinical report that showed he had very high blood pressure. Despite being on three drugs, his blood pressure was 160/110, relatively high for his age. He said, 'I am just thirty-six, and I am too young to have high blood pressure. But my mother has BP, too, you know. I am just like her.'

I did not pay much attention to this seemingly trivial comparison, until he actually went through his first session of regression. Strange as it may appear, there was indeed a link between his health condition and his constant comparison of himself with his mother.

During the session, the young man moved back in time when he was in the womb of his mother in his current life. As a three- or four-month-old foetus in the womb, he heard his father scolding and hitting his pregnant mother. In response, his mother did not utter a word; instead, she swallowed her anger and did not let it out. Consequently, the baby in the womb, and now my client, also learnt how to suppress anger by keeping quiet. He went on to recollect another incident of his father hitting his mother when he was three years old. Yet again, he saw his mother keeping quiet. The tender child automatically was conditioned to deal with anger by suppressing it and not letting it out. As he grew up and started working, he faced many stressful situations with his peers and colleagues, but instead of venting out his anger at being hurt by others, like his mother, he kept suppressing his feelings, time and again.

It is common knowledge that blood pressure rises when a person is angry, but it comes back to normal once the emotion passes. It is a natural and physiological process quite similar to what happens to our BP when we run fast, slow down gradually, and finally come to a halt. However, when any negative emotion like anger is suppressed over time, tension builds up and accumulates in the body, the blood vessels stiffen and modify to control the pressure, which manifests as hypertension. My young client had been facing stressful situations in his office since the past two years, without giving his anger and hurt any vent and thinking that he was *just like his mother*. The tension that he had been holding on to for the last two years, finally took a toll on his health and manifested as hypertension.

Both these cases broadened my perspective to the nuances of mental conditioning. The sources of such conditioning could be multiple—an oath taken in the past, self-conditioning, or being conditioned by the environment—but the effect it has on our health is quite drastic. These are classic examples of mental conditioning that occur by taking an oath or allowing oneself to be conditioned to think in a particular way. These have repercussions on our health. It's like spending a fortune to buy a fully loaded Mercedes car and abusing it for the next ten years by not servicing or maintaining it. To live under the belief that a Mercedes cannot spoil is simple foolishness. *Every matter needs some kind of maintenance.* How am I maintaining my body? How much stress am I giving it? That's why I prefer to term these chronic conditions as 'mindset diseases'—a physical manifestation of the way the mind has been set long ago.

How do we rectify this? *The one tool that each of us has at our disposal no matter what circumstances we are born in, is our will.* Once I understand that I chose to be the way I am, I can firmly decide that I no longer want to remain so and exercise my will to change my current situation. For example, I may have genes that slow my metabolic rate and I put on weight very fast. But once I understand why I chose to be born with this kind of genetic make-up, I can make a firm will to rectify my current situation by regulating my diet, eating healthy food, avoiding sweets and junk, and exercising regularly.

That's exactly what I help my clients with during regression therapy—to break the mental pattern they have created. In fact, the reversal happens automatically when the person is guided to realise that what they are suffering today is a result of a simple oath that they took or a conditioning they allowed themselves to be subjected to many, many years or even lifetimes ago. I guide them to identify the part of the body where they feel the charge of the oath and help them to let it out. As they let out the emotion, the energy and the will that backs it up, including the charge or effect of the oath, is released from the body, bringing them a sense of deep relief.

Often, certain situations may trigger the memory of the oath again. All that I tell my clients to do then is to assert firmly to themselves that 'No, this is a different time. I'm no longer the same person that I was in the past. I'm a different person.' And when they keep reasserting every time, the problem stops bothering them and leaves them forever, because, by then, a new neuropathway is formed. The flow of their thinking changes; they are diverted from a negative path, and within three to six months or sometimes even a year, a positive path flows. A new neuronal connection is formed, a new synapse is formed, new connections are formed, and soon the new condition becomes spontaneous—a part of their very nature. How long it takes for this change to set in permanently depends on how much they have abused their body, their remodelling capacity, and the stage of life that they are in for the tissues, because regenerative ability declines with age. This modality of healing is valid for everyone.

So, during the time of reintegration after regression, I guided my forty-five-year-old client suffering from diabetes to break the mental pattern that he had formed as a young boy. The core emotions that were backing his oath were anger and insecurity. There was anger towards his father for not helping him out with his broken specs, and insecurity that he may have to beg and stretch his hands in front of others if he didn't have enough money.

As a first step, I guided my client to see the reason for his father's denial clearly. As he understood that his father had really wanted to help him, but was under heavy debt and had no money to buy his son a new pair of specs, his anger towards him slowly vanished. Next, I made the young lad of twelve look at himself as a forty-five-year-old man—how materially successful and secure he was—and that was a big revelation for him, which helped in clearing his fear and insecurity. He immediately calmed down with the realisation that he need not fear not making enough money, as he already had so much that even if he considered quitting his job, he could still spend the rest of his life comfortably on his earnings till now. When I reviewed him a month later, he exhibited very positive energy. He said he was able to work much better; in fact, he was excelling more than before as now he felt free of fear or insecurity. Over a period of time, he started sleeping better, and his sugar and BP came under control with the same medication.

In the case of the thirty-six-year-old professional, as he realised that he was not in the shadow of his mother anymore, and as he learnt to deal with anger by expressing it and letting go, his BP normalised. Of course, it took three months for the blood pressure to come down, and he is still on two of the three drugs that he was earlier prescribed.

Our thoughts affect our emotions, and in turn, our emotions disturb the natural flow of positive energy in our body. A disturbance in the flow of such energy in our body ultimately manifests as a physical problem. Through regression therapy, we are able to derive the wisdom of the source of negative thoughts, which create such disturbing emotions. Once we realise what is actually manifesting, we have the ability to change our thinking pattern and bid goodbye to the negative emotion permanently. We can acknowledge the wonderful tool of willpower that we are gifted with and apply it positively to change the environment around our genes and control them. By using our will, we are defining our genes. People may be born with cancer-causing genes, yet they survive the disease—that is the play of epigenetics. The simple understanding that we derive is that our genes do not always create our destiny; we are not only our genes. We can change our destiny very well by using our willpower to control our genes, by changing their environment. *Will is the energy that backs up epigenetics.*

All said and done, the question of healing or rectifying a particular situation or condition comes into the picture only when there is something "wrong" or is not meant to be. But what if we are able to, in the first place, avoid creating such situations for ourselves? It certainly needs a high level of alertness and heightened consciousness to lead a life fully aware of the effects of our thoughts, words and deeds.

I am reminded of an incident where one night, I negligently left the bathroom tap slightly open. However, the next morning I was relieved of a likely guilt of wasting the precious resource when I saw the empty bucket underneath the tap, now almost full of water. Water had trickled down the tap throughout the night, drop by drop, and every single little drop counted in filling up the whole bucket. I could draw a parallel from this principle to what we suffer today. *Every single drop counts.*

The best way to help ourselves is to let go of our patterns of thinking and acting, which we often hold on to for any reason whatsoever, daily. Some of these chronic diseases may have roots in our genetic make-up, but largely, they manifest due to a fixed mindset over some time. In such cases, the only thing I have to say is: *Let go.*

The Power of the Subconscious
Mental Conditioning Behind the Physical Condition

If someone were to ask me the exact time when epigenetics come into play in a person's life, I would reply unhesitatingly, 'From the time of conception in the mother's womb.' Cultural and traditional ideologies apart, there is plenty of proven research to conclude that the mother's state of mind and emotions directly impact the child in her womb.

Many of my clients have revealed that they experience tremendous trauma when faced with any sort of negative information from their immediate environment, which, in turn, affects the baby in the womb. The cause of the trauma could be a friend, family member, or sometimes even the doctor attending on the pregnant woman.

One of the most dramatic cases of trauma in my experience was when a doctor thoughtlessly disclosed to a mother who had done an ultrasound scan during her pregnancy, 'Your baby is not going to be normal. Come back after two days: we shall repeat the scan to confirm the findings.'

For the next two days, the expecting mother literally went through hell. The best part was that after two days when the scan was repeated, the doctor's earlier findings were confirmed negative! The growing child in the womb was stated to be normal.

However, the damage had already been done during the interval between the two scans—on the tender foetus through the mother's extremely worried mental state.

Subsequently, as the child is delivered into the world, she/he is susceptible to the direct environment, unlike the indirect conditioning through the mother while in the womb. Society, religion, cultural values and beliefs and the mother's own personality—all of these play a role; and the physical ramifications of such mental conditioning is beyond imagination. Healing occurs through regression when the client goes back in time, understands the truth and becomes open to freeing himself or herself from the bonds of such mental conditioning.

In my experience, the strongest conditioning of people happens through their parents—and the public at large. I keep revisiting the insights that I have gained from such parental and mass conditioning as strategic bits of knowledge that broaden my vision and understanding of the mind's power and the subconscious.

The Impact of Parental Conditioning

'Doctor, I ate two ice creams yesterday! I knew I was going to catch a cold ...' stated a toddler solemnly, as she walked into my cabin with her even more solemn parents.

This is a common scenario that I encounter during my paediatric practice—90 per cent of the parents bring their children with complaints such as, 'Yesterday, he had a cold drink and, look, this morning he has woken up with cough, cold and fever!' My attempts at trying to make the concerned parents understand that all diseases—including the common cold—have an incubation period of a few days to a week, often go in vain. I persistently tell them that a cold drink consumed twelve hours ago cannot result in an onslaught of the common cold and its associated symptoms. However, it all falls on deaf ears.

I have noted that sooner or later, the children start aping their parents by repeating the same dialogue, and saving them the trouble of explaining how the cold set in! These observations inevitably turn my attention to the science of parental conditioning.

Studies of brainwaves in adults and children have highlighted the importance of the subconscious mind in the development of children, the most important phase being between the birth of the child and the age of six. During this time span, the subconscious mind has the ability to download enormous amounts of information. EEG readings of children demonstrate that during the first two years of life, a child's brain is in the lowest EEG frequency range called delta, and afterwards, it increases and operates in the frequency of the theta range. These brain wave patterns, which are so slow, signify that children under the age of six are functioning below consciousness, that is, their subconscious mind is very much active.

In layman's terms, below this age, they are in a state of hypnotic trance. This allows the child's observations of his surroundings, his perceptions of the world, and experiences of life to be downloaded directly into the subconscious. All of the information goes directly into the subconscious without any discrimination, filtering or analysis. And given that the subcortical centres of the brain can process 40 billion bits of information per second (as opposed to the cortex that processes 40 bits per second), children below six, in all their innocence, rapidly download a powerful amount of unfiltered data into their subconscious.

This is a big concern for me as a paediatrician and a parent, for this time of raw learning sets the foundation for our habits and behaviours, which is 95 per cent of who we are as adults. This subconscious learning determines how we think, act and feel in the years to come. It dictates our personality, and, after all, personality creates our personal reality. The advances in neurosciences have helped me to understand the critical role that we as adults can play in the development and moulding of children during the first six years of their life when their minds are still tender or in a state of hypnotic trance; when they spend their maximum time mixing their imaginary world with the real world. The information that reaches their subconscious mind forms the foundation for the way in which they perceive the world, their beliefs, and ultimately their success and, most importantly, their well-being.

——

Five-year-old Mona was my very first paediatric case in regression. She walked into my clinic with a very inquisitive look on her face, hand-in-hand with her young mother. Thick, heavy glasses rested on her little nose, and I couldn't help wondering how awful it looked on her otherwise cute and innocent face. Her mother looked very anxious and sad. She said,

'My daughter has such beautiful eyes, but these glasses make them look so horrible.' She explained that the child was diagnosed with Hypermetropia.

Hypermetropia is an eye disorder more commonly known as farsightedness or long-sightedness. It is a condition that results in blurry vision of nearby objects, while objects that are far away appear normal.

On interacting with Mona, I found her to be very sweet and talkative, with a willingness to cooperate and do as she was told. Yet the first thoughts that came to my mind were, 'Will I really be able to help this girl through regression? After all, her condition could very well be genetic. She might have been born with the defect, which was diagnosed later than sooner.'

My initial hesitation to treat her was influenced by my mind schooled in allopathy. But on closer examination of her case history, I discovered that her father had mild myopia, and as her mother was free of any eye disorder, she did not wear any eyeglasses. Thus, it was clear that the girl's vision could not be linked to her family history.

I decided to go ahead with regression, assuring the mother that it was a simple process through which we would try to find the cause of her daughter's problem. At the same time, I also cautioned her that I could not guarantee a successful result. If at all the disorder was genetic, in all probability, Mona's regression would not reveal anything substantial to identify the root cause of her defective eyesight. Asking the mother to wait outside the room, I started chatting with the girl who was more than willing to participate.

Since I was dealing with a child for the first time, I had to use a different approach to induce her into a trance. Usually, most of my adult clients take a while to go into a deep state of trance, where they are able to access their subconscious. But with Mona's session, and with those of other children that followed, I came to realise that children were much more amenable and mouldable than their adult counterparts. It was easier to take children into a state of trance and have them tap into their subconscious.

Nevertheless, I was dealing with a child and I knew it was better to talk her language to make my work simpler. I told her, 'Let's play a game—a game that has a lot to do with your mind. Your mind is so strong and powerful that it can help you find the problem with your eyes. Are you willing to play with me? If you win, I shall give you a little gift.'

Mona was excited and more than willing to join the fun. I went on to explain the rules: 'Throughout the game, you need to keep your eyes closed and follow my instructions. You may share with me whatever you experience, whatever you go through, when your eyes are closed.' The girl sat on the couch and I asked her to close her eyes. Within two minutes of suggestions, she was in a state of trance.

> Me: Connect with your eyes. Go deep, deep, deep to understand where the problem lies. When and where did the issue with your eyes begin?

Mona: I am small. I am watching my favourite cartoon on TV.

Me: How old are you?

Mona: I'm small. I can walk.

I gathered she was recollecting the time when she was one or two years old.

Me: How are you feeling watching the cartoon?

Mona: Oh, I feel so nice!

I was amused by the gleeful smile on her face, as she enjoyed a recap of her favourite programme on TV.

Mona: The cartoon characters are so funny! I like it….

I gave her the pause to allow her to cherish the memory. Suddenly, she assumed an agitated tone.

Mona: Mumma is coming and telling me, 'You're watching too much TV. Your eyes will get spoiled.'

And from her state of trance, I heard the child imitating a powerful suggestion from her mother. *If you watch TV, your eyes will spoil.* And it left such an impact on the girl's mind that whenever she would sit to watch television, the thought that her eyes will spoil would already be at work in her subconscious.

As Mona recollected this suggestion from her mom, she started rubbing her eyes.

Me: Why are you rubbing your eyes?

Mona: They feel tired, so I'm rubbing them. I am scared that my eyes will spoil. Mumma said if I watch TV too much, my eyes will spoil.

I could see that each time she sat to watch TV, her subconscious mind would throw up the suggestion that 'Oh, my eyes will get spoiled.' She would keep rubbing her eyes and unconsciously keep making the suggestion she had heard from her mother to herself. Sadly, the mother had no clue about the damage her seemingly harmless statement had done to her daughter's tender mind, finally resulting in her eye disorder.

Once, I was able to identify the root of her problem, I had to assume an altogether different approach to initiate the process of integration in the child. I asked her a few more questions.

Me: Who are your best friends?

Mona mentioned three names.

Me: Do they wear glasses?

Mona: No, none of them wear glasses.

Me: Do they watch TV?

Mona: Oh yes, they do!

Me: For how long in a day?

Mona: I do not know exactly, but they certainly spend more hours in front of the TV than I do. I know that because they keep telling me about all the different programmes they get to watch on TV!

Me: Did their eyes spoil? Do they wear glasses?

Mona: No, they don't wear glasses.

Me: So then why do you think your eyes will spoil? You don't seem to watch TV for long hours.

Mona: You are right ... Compared to my friends, I watch less TV. My eyes should be better!

Me: Good. Now connect with your eyes and tell them firmly that you do not watch TV for long hours. That there is no reason why your eyes alone should spoil when all your friends are happy with good eyesight.

Mona: Okay ... I see a brown patch in each eye.

Me: What do you want to do with those brown patches?

Mona: I want to remove them.

Me: Go ahead, remove those patches. How do they look?

Mona: They look like mud. They look bad; I want to throw them out.

Me: Who is stopping you? Throw the dirty mud out of your eyes and instead fill them with a nice blue light.

I was amazed by the young girl's willingness to cooperate and the creative potential of her imaginative mind. It was as if she was performing a mental surgery on her own eyes, like a professional doctor.

With that, we finished the session. Mona woke up with a cheerful face and a twinkle in her eyes.

Mona: My eyes will definitely become alright....

Me: They will, won't they? Let's wait and watch!

The girl's enthusiasm and positivity was contagious and so I said what I said. But in my heart of hearts, I was not very sure about the success of this case. We were dealing with Hypermetropia here, with eyeglasses of the power of +4.5 degrees. Yet, as per the protocol, after the session, I debriefed Mona's anxious mother on the revelations from her daughter's regression. She was very surprised that one little suggestion of her's had impacted and affected the child's mind to this extent.

In her own defense, she tried to explain, 'My mother would keep saying that television spoils the eyes and hence she would not let us watch TV. Unlike my daughter, I was not affected by my mother's suggestion or saying. So then why did my child get affected to the extent that her eyes were spoiled?' I could understand her confusion. I explained to her that every child is unique. *Children have a mindset of their own; they think and process information differently from each other.*

After three months when Mona came for a follow-up, her mother brought me the happy tidings that her daughter's eye power had gone down to +3.5 from +4.5. This news was very reassuring and encouraging to me, all at the same time. In light of these positive developments, I suggested a mental exercise to be undertaken by Mona twice a day. I told the mother to ask her daughter to close her eyes and imagine blue light filling them up and the brown patches vanishing completely. I suggested she do this exercise mentally every night before going to bed and also each morning soon after waking up.

By the end of one year, Mona's eye power had come down to +1 and it continues to be so till today. This was indeed one of the most astonishing cases I had handled so far, and I was once again bowled over by the power of suggestion, the power of the subconscious. It was amazing how effectively and successfully an innocent child could heal herself simply by the power of thought.

——

Everyone, however, may not be as lucky as the young girl with Hypermetropia. For, sometimes, childhood conditioning can mar (or make) the person's whole life, as it happened in the case of my forty-eight-year-old client, who had been living a very lonely life ever since her divorce ten years ago. The first time I met her I could sense that she was very disturbed, with a fear of the future, and unable to form new relationships, resulting in frustration with life. When I dug up her history during our conversation, I found out that her relationship with her husband hadn't worked out well, plainly because of her disinterest in sex. Physical intercourse with her husband had never been a pleasurable act for her; it had always been painful. As a result, her husband had left her feeling badly rejected, saying, 'We are not meant to be with each other.'

During her regression, the first memory that presented itself was when she was playing with a boy as a little girl of six or seven years old. She recollected her mom warning her, 'It's not good to play with boys, be careful.' The little girl was surprised, but kept quiet. Then another memory came up: she was eleven years old and had just attained puberty. She again recounted her mother talking to her about sex and referring to it as a terrible act: 'Look, you're turning into a woman now. Sex is horrible. It can make you pregnant, it can get you diseases. So stay away from boys!' The girl froze listening to her mother's words, which created a deep impression in her subconscious mind.

Next, she went back to a memory when she was thirteen years old and was trying to get intimate with a boy. As soon as he started touching her, she pushed him away and walked away with the fear that she would get pregnant or acquire some disease. With time, these fears kept building inside her. However, at the age of sixteen and under the influence of her friends, she chucked aside all that her mother had told her about sex and gave it a try. Fatefully, it turned out to be very painful and terrible for her! Needless to say, she concluded, 'My mother was right: sex is a very painful thing.' Since then, she could never enjoy sex, which ultimately ended in broken relationships in the future.

When I dug deeper as to why the mother carried such feelings, I found that she had been abused sexually when she was a teenager. I was fascinated and, at the same time, a little sad, when I realised how a particular conditioning of the mind gets transferred across generations. In the case of my forty-eight-year-old client, her entire life was marred because of such conditioning. At the start of her sessions, I discovered that she carried a latent hatred for her mother. When she came to know that her mother had been sexually abused, her hatred went away at the time of integration through reasoning. But all said and done, she was still not happy with what her mother had done to her—it had cost her a lifetime.

This knowledge of children learning through their subconscious mind, in the absence of analytical abilities to process what they see or hear, gave me a new understanding of the connection between their physical body, mind and soul.

- The child's awareness is on their internal environment; they easily notice changes in how they feel inside.

- When they feel differently inside, it perks their attention to the giver or sender of the information—and that creates a memory.
- There are bugs inside our body all the time. If the subconscious mind downloads a link between drinking or eating cold food and falling sick, through repeated exposure to that idea or suggestion, the mind-body connection turns on the existing bugs and there is a reaction caused by such conditioning of the subconscious mind.

The same formula applies when children watch a particular programme repeatedly on TV. They start mimicking the character without any discrimination, because they have mirror neurons (empathy neurons) that turn on the same circuit in the brains as if they are actually doing it.

——

Once a couple came in with the concern that their son had become very violent, to the extent that he would even hit others. They complained that, of late, he had also been throwing a lot of unreasonable tantrums and demanding things to be bought and given to him whenever they would go out, irrespective of whether he needed them or not. While giving their child's history, the parents asserted that he had not been exposed to any violence either at home or school. As I kept enquiring, I realised that the boy had been watching a lot of TV, especially one particular animated programme featuring a child superhero whose only aim was to bash up all evil in the world. I was amused to discover that this boy had actually been aping his favourite television character, and was sincerely beating up people whenever he would observe something 'bad' or 'wrong' happening.

Interestingly, as the boy visited his memory of watching the programme, I observed his body becoming very stiff on the recliner. His parents confirmed that it was exactly how his body would be when he was actually watching TV at home! Moreover, his regression revealed that even the advertisements that were played during the intervals had left a deep impact on his subconscious. As a result, whenever the boy went to a mall or a shop, he would insist his parents buy the things that he was regularly watching on the television.

As soon as the parents realised the cause for their child's erratic behaviour, they diverted him from spending time in front of the TV by coaxing him to play outdoors and spending quality time with him by engaging in other constructive activities. Soon they were able to observe a significant improvement in their son's temperament and behaviour.

We don't realise the intensity of the impact gadgets produce on children's minds. I find them getting very angry with their parents when they don't give them the iPad or mobile phone, or let them sit at the desktop or things like that. It's very scary. I call it 'gadgetomania', because these children are going crazy for gadgets. And it is we who give these gadgets to them, because we don't have time for them; we're so busy. In the process, we don't realise what we are doing with our child's brain, which is still growing. It's very important what and how we convey or suggest to our children, for their moulding and thinking depends on it. This calls for conscious parenting, especially in today's times, as our words and the vibes they carry and the environment that we expose the little ones to, have the deepest impact on their tender minds.

Cancer in a New Light

I once undertook a pilot study, with 100 healthy people free from any sort of ailment as the sample population. I asked each of them, 'What is the first thing that comes to your mind when you hear the word 'cancer'?' Ninety of them instantly said 'death' and the rest replied with either 'pain' or 'suffering'. Today, with the onslaught of the media, a lot of negativity is created and connected with cancer.

It is not only my hunch, but my conviction that in the earlier centuries, when we did not know much about the disease, we lived longer and happier in spite of contracting the illness. No wonder ignorance is bliss!

Most of the cancer cases that came to me for regression were already in the fourth stage. The one thing that struck me as being common to all of them was the way the news of the disease was disclosed to them by their physicians. The moment of diagnosis was so pivotal, as if with the news, a death-timer was set up for the suffering patient. I have generally observed that at the time of hearing the diagnosis, the power of the mind comes into play, which sets the ball rolling for the disease to either progress or regress.

The trauma doesn't end with the doctor disclosing: 'You have cancer, you have only six months to live,' but it continues; for once the news about the ailment spreads, even the people around start looking at you with pity and sympathy: 'Oh, the poor girl is going to die.' The vibes sent from the environment are worse, and the poor patient is as good as dead that moment, rather than waiting for the next six months! Such mass conditioning can be very devastating, and personally, I feel, is an important cause for the excessive fear associated with cancer.

Other factors play a role too. From the individual point of view, each time we consume a drug for cancer, we inevitably do so with the thought of the disease at the back of our minds. If there are any other health complications, we may take it as an additional blow or setback solely meant to aggravate the existing cancer. So, now on the one hand, we have the play of mass conditioning, while on the other, in today's digital world where we have unlimited access to all types of information, at the back of our minds, there is a latent fear brewing that our lifestyles, our choices and our environments are slowly leading us to our doom. Another interesting thing to observe is that two people may be living in the same environment and may have the same physical immunity, but one succumbs to cancer and the other doesn't. Why is that so?

Ultimately, when we delve into the root of this disease, I feel it cannot be traced to any single cause; there are multiple factors that need consideration. The person's soul *karma,* genetic predisposition, environment and lifestyle, and the way the mind has been conditioned to think—all matter and play a role. However, if I have to determine an important factor in the outcome of cancer, I would, without hesitation, hold the person's mindset as the important determinant, especially the fear and predisposition to the idea that a diagnosis of cancer results in death.

When we think negatively, we attract all negativity that ultimately weakens our resolve and cooperation. It is finally the mind that decides. If we firmly decide, 'Enough is enough. I have closely observed my life; I know why I am suffering. I've learnt my lesson and now I choose to let go,' I am confident that the very disease we dread can bring about a U-turn in life for good! Accepting it and undergoing the latest available treatment with this intent is an important determinant in the outcome of the disease.

The work with my cancer patients has led me so far to address their mindset; facilitating a shift in their thinking, allowing them to accept their illness actively, and in the process, fostering positivity. When the disease has advanced to the final stage, freedom from fear may be the closest substitute for the joy of recovery. During the sessions, my clients gain an understanding of what had gone wrong in their lives that ultimately brought them cancer, what unnecessary memory they had been holding on to, and the cause for any kind of negative emotion that they had been carrying since long.

Positive emotions do not produce any kind of disease, let alone cancer; it is primarily negative emotions like fear, guilt, sadness, anger, and vengeance, which are deeply embedded in our subconscious, that ultimately manifest in our physical body. Though most of my clients succumbed to cancer, the upside was that through regression they were able to see the disease in a new light, embrace it wholeheartedly and take it within their stride to make the most of whatever life was left in their hands. In some cases, the turnaround involved stepping out of toxic relationships, quitting stressful jobs, changing their home environment, and resorting to seeking a higher purpose and meaning in life.

One of my colleagues who extensively works with cancer patients shared a very encouraging observation:

> 'The few people who I think have progressed in a broader sense, in spite of their cancer, are people who've really looked at this disease as a transformative moment. Immediately upon hearing the diagnosis they may have felt low and considered it to be a diagnosis of death. But when we begin to coach them and work with them, we realise that if we can take them into a space where they start thinking of the disease as a harbinger of transformation, they are able to strike gold. They begin by putting away sour relationships, and change jobs and homes. Some of them even leave their abusive husbands and move on to find loving partners.'

——

A thirty-two-year-old gentleman presented a history of brain tumour, which he was diagnosed with in 2012 when he had a seizure and fell unconscious. A scan revealed a tumour close to his speech centre, and he was operated on for it soon after diagnosis. Thereafter, he underwent radiotherapy sessions, and a repeat of the scan showed regression of the tumour.

However, one day in September 2017, he had a strange experience. He suddenly felt as if he was choking and was not able to express himself verbally. He mentioned there was a gap of at least fifteen seconds from his ideation to expression. He felt compelled to undergo a scan and just as he had dreaded, it revealed a recurrence of the brain tumour.

When I asked him about his reaction the first time he was diagnosed with the tumour, he said he was just shocked, but not scared. But at its recurrence, he was shocked, and at the same time, had also felt sad, because he now had a child to look after. I probed further to understand if anything had drastically gone wrong in the last one year, and he revealed that he had been suffering from disturbed sleep and a lot of stress both towards his work and family. That was the cue I was waiting for, and I decided to explore deeper into the roots of his concern through regression.

As my client relaxed on the recliner, I firmly suggested, 'Connect with the swelling in your brain. Go deeper and bring out what's stuck in there. What's growing there?' He replied, 'There's something black—a lot of anger.' I prompted him to dig deeper, and he moved back in time when he had just got married.

It was the year 2012. Right from the start, there seemed to be a lot of misunderstandings between him and his wife, which would often end up with him being physically violent with her. The primary cause for the misunderstanding was that he would support his parents instead of listening to his wife. She would inevitably feel miserable and fight with him, and he, in turn, would get physical to stop her. However, later he would end up feeling guilty for his actions, especially when he realised that his parents were more at fault than his own wife.

One peculiar observation I could make was the presence of a strong feeling deep in his mind that 'No matter how much I try to speak or convey, I am not understood. Neither does my wife understand nor does my mother.' He regressed to a moment when he was so angry that he actually poured boiling milk on his own head to stop his wife's yelling, because he was not able to speak out or express his point. He was not able to pacify her with his words, and the domestic violence only got worse.

Just about a year before he was diagnosed with the tumour, he recounted himself taking an oath after a big fight at home: 'I am so tired of these fights. I am not heard or understood, so I will not fight with anyone anymore, no matter what happens.'

After that, even though he felt angry and miserable, he would suppress his anger and not express anything. This was a clear insight into to how the guilt and anger suppressed deep inside him were probably causing the tumour in his brain. Surprisingly, the tumour was near his speech centre—a metaphor for his inability to speak and express himself—and that was the connecting link between his subconscious and physical manifestation, which was brought out through regression.

When I reviewed him one month later, he said that he felt much lighter and did not feel any suppressed anger towards his wife. He was no longer holding on to his vow and was able to express his feelings and ideas more calmly than ever before. However, longer follow-ups are still needed to see what actually happens to the tumour in his brain.

--

In some of the advanced nations of the West, it is mandatory to disclose the diagnosis, prognosis and treatment plan to the patient's face. The good part here in India is that—and I prefer this approach—even in some of the leading hospitals, half of the time, some of the older patients don't even know they have cancer. They come with their family for treatment and the family members are told. They die in a much better state of mind and situation, because they have not feared the disease during their lifetime.

My appeal to the medical fraternity is not to prognosticate, because every individual is unique. We calculate a survival period for a specific patient of cancer, based on a general study of a large population, beyond which there are sure to be survivors of even terminal cases! So how can the same prognosis hold true for everybody?

Instead, how about stressing on the positives? For example, we can say: 'We don't know how the disease will take a turn inside you, because every individual is unique. People have different immunities, different genetic-patterns, their living conditions vary, and how each responds to chemotherapy is also different. So, we really cannot predict. But we can assure you that there are plenty of people who have lived through it and have been cured of cancer.'

At any given point in time, I would always insist that if the family can handle it well, do not disclose to the patient that they have cancer. If at all it needs to be conveyed, do so in a very positive way, in a very conducive environment, for after all, epigenetics never misses a chance to play its role.

In my life, I have known people surviving cancer plainly by using their willpower to live. Having understood the root of the disease, they firmly condition their minds to change the environment around themselves and let go of whatever they are holding on to in their subconscious, which is the root of manifesting cancer. I look at them as warriors, capable of changing their destiny purely by their act of will.

The Cord of Love
Regression in Children Through Surrogacy

I always trust the instinct of the mother. Even in children who can articulate their feelings well, I reach out to the mother for her observations and her gut instinct, for she is the only one who can connect the dots. The deep invisible connection that exists between a mother and child mesmerises me. This point was driven home when I became a parent myself.

My wife and I were watching our two-year-old boy having fun on the playground, when my wife mentioned with some concern that she felt he was beginning to develop a fever. The physician in me immediately dismissed it as the symptoms simply did not add up. Sure enough, a few hours later, he was burning with fever. Instead of snapping back at me with an 'I told you so', my wife silenced me with her intuition and premonition about our little son's health.

A cord of energy deeply connects the mother and her child. While the umbilical cord is there for all to see and reaffirms this nourishing connection, the emotional cord that connects the astral, ethereal, or subtle bodies of the mother and child is a forgotten science. This cord allows for the exchange of emotional or etheric energy between the two beings. These invisible channels determine the characteristics and nature of the visible physical relationships. Unknown to myself, I was to use this understanding of the etheric bond between mother and child in healing a population of patients that I am fondest of: children.

Now, the primary requisite to go through a regression session is to be able to close your eyes and sit quietly for an extended period of time. So how to regress a child who could not close his eyes and sit still even for a few moments? This was the dilemma that I faced when, for the very first time, a desperate mother came to consult me on her six-year-old autistic child. While talking and listening to her, all of a sudden, the incident on the playground with my wife and son flashed before my eyes and an idea came to my mind. I asked the mother if she was willing to try an experiment with me. *Would she be willing to help her child heal by being his surrogate during the regression?* The mother was more than willing to do anything for her son, and that became the first case of surrogate regression that I handled successfully.

The word 'surrogate', derived from the Latin word '*surrogatus*', is defined in the dictionary as 'elect as a substitute'. In this method of surrogate regression, I use one of the parents, either the mother or the father, as a substitute to heal the child. My conviction and experience in the energy bonds between the subtle bodies of the mother and child was the scientific basis for the experiment that I conducted for the first time in 2011. The details are provided in the latter half of this chapter.

While facilitating regression therapy in children by using their parents as surrogates, I have observed that the ones who benefit the most are the parents themselves. First and foremost, an understanding of the reasons for their child's present life brings them immense relief and stems guilt. With such an understanding, they no longer operate from fear but can tap into the inherent love that they carry for their child. The child is accepted for its choice of living life in this particular way with a lot of love. This fundamental change in understanding acts as a catalyst in changing the dynamics of the parent-child relationship and it improves the quality of every minute of the life to be lived ahead.

As I was assimilating this technique of surrogate regression for young children who cannot express themselves, I was presented with an opportunity to explore further. A three-year-old was not meeting the basic developmental milestones—he could speak only two-three words but had a good ability to comprehend. He suffered from hypotonia in his lower limbs (also called floppy baby syndrome, causing very low muscular strength/tone in limbs). The clinical diagnosis was a genetic mutation[1] that caused an intense developmental delay. In the view of clinicians, this was a permanent disability, which would require the child to be managed with therapy and care-giving.

While taking the child's birth history, the mother revealed some intriguing details about her pregnancy and delivery.

> Mother: The ultrasonography report at seven months of my pregnancy was shattering: it revealed some kind of disability in the child. The doctor said that I was carrying a very handicapped baby. The news devastated me, and I remained in that state of shock for the next few days. Strangely, after a few days, the doctor called and said that they would like to conduct one more scan to reconfirm the findings of the earlier sonography. The second scan rendered the findings of the first one void. The doctor reassured me that my baby would be normal. But I couldn't help worrying even after that.
>
> My son was born nineteen days later than the due date. I was very keen to have a normal delivery and, therefore, wouldn't have minded waiting for a few days more. But the doctor was afraid that they wouldn't be able to save the baby if they delayed the delivery any further and so insisted that I go in for a cesarean (LSCS). I had no option but to agree.

The child had indeed been born normal, but with time, they found that he was not developing according to the usual growth milestones. The parents, out of concern, consulted a doctor who confirmed delayed development in the child. At the time of history-taking, the anxious mother revealed a strange observation about her son: she felt as if his legs were as hard as rocks and that there seemed to be something stuck in his sacrum. This was quite intriguing from the perspective of regression and we decided to explore this observation.

I started the session using the mother as a surrogate for her child. Soon she regressed into another lifetime.

> Mother: I see a dark-skinned boy. He seems to be around ten years of age. He looks desolate, standing near a mine of rocks. He is carrying really heavy rocks down the hill. His back seems to be hurting and his legs are shaking. He is my son in my present life.
>
> There is a snake … It looks like the boy is trying to avoid it … He slips and falls, causing the rocks to slide. A large rock falls on his legs, crushing them badly. The boy is unable to move. He lies there in that state for quite some time, until a man comes along and takes him home.

I nudge my client to go back further in that lifetime for more details on this strange boy.

> Mother: The boy is seven years old and they call him Sikhal. It looks like the 20th century, a marshy village land somewhere in the north of India. Sikhal's mother has passed away while delivering his little sister. The father is an alcoholic and irresponsible. He cares the least for his children. For a year, the villagers take care of the children, and afterwards, the chief of the village decides to hand them over to their relatives.
>
> The uncle and aunt, in whose custody Sikhal and his sister are now in, do not treat them kindly. They take advantage of their situation and sell the children off to the village mine owner to repay their debts. Sikhal works hard, and his daily chore is to carry heavy rocks. The only thought that keeps him going is that 'I have to be there for my sister. There is no one else to take care of her. I will work hard, come what may, and take care of her.'
>
> It is during his routine back-breaking manual work, one day, that he sees a snake. He panics and slips. A rock slides crushing both his back and his legs. The younger sister looks on helplessly.

A Samaritan finds the children and takes them home, but Sikhal dies after a few days.

I asked my surrogate client if she could make out the thought in Sikhal's mind at the time of dying.

> Mother: The worry for his three-year-old sister is the predominant thought in him as he passes on. The little girl, on her part, is not able to express anything. She loved her brother ... I love my brother ... I want him back....

As the mother experienced this, she began to sob with the realisation that she was personally intertwined with this boy from the past, who was her handicapped son in the present. *She had been Sikhal's younger sister in that lifetime and he had passed on while worrying about her!* We felt the need to explore further to gain an understanding on the deep attachment the little sister felt towards her brother. The mother moved further back in time, to yet another life in the past.

> Mother: It's a tribal fishing hamlet, I think, in Thailand. I am a crab-seller. Life in this village is all about survival. I am the mother of a healthy grown-up boy, and I am seven months pregnant with another child. It's time for the delivery of this child, and I am surrounded by the older tribal women of the village who are helping in the delivery.
> The baby has come out. It's a boy. The women who are surrounding me suddenly start commenting that the child looks very frail. Some even suggest abandoning him as they were sure he would not live long. I am shell-shocked and shaken by their taunts and comments. I resolve not to give up and do everything in my power to make my son thrive.
> My son grows up never to walk. Instead, he moves about crawling on his belly like a salamander. He is very talented, with a mesmerising voice and fine articulation. He goes on to become a fantastic crab-seller—one of the best in the hamlet.
> One day, sensing that he has some nutrition deficiency, the boy crawls into the sea and finds a particular variety of seaweed

that he somehow knows to have the ability to cure his deficiency. Not only his but others' too—the weed has healing properties. He dries the seaweed and sells it to people, convincing them about its health benefits with his beautiful articulation. People of the hamlet rush to buy the weed from my son: they realise it has some very important minerals to keep the body healthy.

Soon, with his talent and by selling the seaweed, the boy becomes rich and I, as his mother, am very proud of him. I die feeling very secure and satisfied about the abilities of my crippled son, who is now almost seventeen years of age, to lead a successful and independent life.

A vision of this life gave my surrogate client a lot of hope. In the current life, her biggest worry that 'My son will not be able to endure and overcome his challenges and make something good out of his life' was replaced with an assurance that 'Though my son's development is delayed, he will surely overcome his challenges and make good of his life.'

Two days after this session, an ecstatic mother called to report: 'A miracle has happened. He has started rubbing and massaging his legs. He thumped his feet on the ground to feel it, took our hands (one on each side) and walked! He normally walks by holding onto things but never felt secure enough to only hold our hands. This is huge progress!' I was stunned, unable to match the mother's elation. She had been able to help the child let go of the memory from his legs of falling down and being crushed while serving as a surrogate.

Despite seeing these transformative events being played out repeatedly in my clinic, with client after client, the boy's leg movements just after two days of his surrogate regression were a bit too much for me to digest clinically and scientifically.

I must add here that the parents were super proactive. They took their understanding of the memory and metaphor of the past lives to a much deeper level and helped their child with other physical therapies. They supplemented it with the Anat Baniel

Method (ABM), an exceptional system of movement and learning that is based on the science of brain plasticity[2]. Over a period of six months now, the boy is blooming—running as if chasing a storm!

Yet we needed another session to come full circle. The child's mother was very concerned about her husband and, sure enough, he confided that he was still hopeless, scared, and even devastated when he thought of his son's future. So, this time we regressed into the child's past using the father as a surrogate.

> Father: I see a boy... His name is Urtuk... It's me... The place looks like a village somewhere in Central India. I look happy. I am living with my parents and younger brother.
>
> I am fifteen years old... My mother is crippled and lying on the bed unable to even move. She is suffering. A few months pass. Mother dies... I feel hopeless and helpless... I am not able to help my mother. I am so useless. I seem to be going into a cocoon of despair and shock. I stop all kinds of social interaction. I never marry. It is as if I am stuck in that state of shock, in that feeling of hopelessness. I live until a ripe old age, just sitting outside my hut filled with weariness, sadness and despair.

As my surrogate client—this time the father—looked closer into that lifetime, he found that Urtuk's mother was indeed his son in the present life. The doctor's message about his child's genetic abnormality and the resulting handicap in the current life triggered the memory of the same despair, shock and hopelessness that he had experienced at the loss of his mother in his past life. In the present, he continuously felt pity for his boy and miserable for himself with the thought that, 'I am losing my zest and will to live, as I can't change much for my son. To have an abnormal child is so devastating. It's a big blow to me.'

Through regression, it dawned on him that for the past three and a half years, a strange feeling had been enveloping and bogging him down. This feeling was so intense that despite all the efforts that he was putting towards remedies and cures, he was feeling 'stuck'. Once he had undergone catharsis during regression and had integrated all the information and understanding, the beautiful connection that he shared with his son seeped into him, filling him with warmth and hope.

—-—

In 2011, a desperate mother came to consult me about her six-year-old son who was autistic, hyperactive and prone to bouts of aggression and violence at school. She also conveyed, with profound sadness, that this aggressive behaviour was predominantly towards her; her husband seemed to evoke a very loving side of their son. The boy also had a fear of closing his eyes. 'The best way to help the child is through regression,' I thought. And that became my very first case in surrogate regression.

I began the session by guiding the mother, my surrogate client, to a state of trance. Very soon, she relaxed and with closed eyes, she travelled back in time to the conception of her child. After guiding her to connect to her bonding with her pregnancy and sensing it, I asked her to invite her six-year-old son into that space. Guiding her, I gently nudged her to feel the connection between her and him. She connected with him at three levels: mind, heart, and the navel. I guided her further, 'Tell your child that you are going to work on his behalf, work with him to find out the cause of this problem.'

She moved back in time to when she was four months pregnant. She had been advised bed-rest and had moved to her parents' home for support. Given the length of her confinement and her boredom, she subsequently asked her husband to move in with her. Very soon, he and her father started getting into petty everyday squabbles. These fights made her very edgy, and soon she began to brood: 'It was so peaceful before my husband got here. I am responsible for this mess.'

The brooding began to spiral until she began to think: 'Life was all smooth and happy until I got pregnant with this baby. Damn it! Why did this baby come?' Within a few minutes, she corrected this thinking, as she realised it was no fault of the baby. But the feeling that the baby in the womb was accountable for her misery had been frozen. Feeling this in her subconscious state, she began to cry realising that her baby could have felt her vehement emotions even though they were only for a few fleeting moments.

As part of the therapy, it was important for her to not carry this guilt. So, I asked her to connect with her baby and speak to the child and ask for forgiveness, explaining that she did not mean any of this.

We then went on to explore the reason(s) for her son's aggressive behaviour, and she travelled to a time in her present life when her son was a year old. She was flustered to see him tied tightly to a chair, because even from her state of deep trance, she was absolutely certain that she had never tied him up in that fashion. I guided her to release him from the chair, shower him with affection, and tell him that something had been wrong but it was over now. Even as an observer, I could not comprehend the situation. Slowly, I guided her out of the session.

While the mother was shocked by the episode of blaming her baby in her womb, she was very perplexed by the image of her small child being tied up and his extremely agitated state at being immobile. The answers came when the boy's grandmother owned up to tying him to a chair every morning and evening while she cooked and her daughter (the boy's mother) was away at work. Needless to say, in that state, the child developed extreme frustration and aggressiveness, while trying to be free!

To me, this whole experience of the mother being able to connect and 'see' an incident that she was not a physical part of, was stunning and amazing. I decided to hold all expectations at bay, stay neutral, and observe.

During the review, six weeks after being regressed, the first positive change she reported was that her son had stopped beating her. He had also become less aggressive. Now my scepticism gave way to curiosity and I decided to explore this connection between mother and son.

In the next session, she regressed to a lifetime in Europe in the 1870's where she saw herself falling in love with a man who her father did not approve of. As a result, she severed ties with her father and left home to live with her boyfriend. But unfortunately, when she was five months pregnant with their child, her boyfriend met with an accident and died. For many months thereafter, she was engulfed by an overwhelming loneliness on being estranged from all her loved ones. However, after giving birth to her son, she found solace in her little companion.

But when the child was around the age of one, in that lifetime, she saw him displaying abnormal development. Her doctor confirmed that a lot of intervention would be needed to restore the boy to normalcy, but with no guarantee of success. Being a single mother, consumed first by fear and then with guilt, she left her son at an orphanage and resumed her life. However, she carried the guilt of abandoning the child even to her deathbed. At the time of death, the anguish of abandoning such a small, precious, guiltless child, made her invite the same soul into her next life as her child, so she could pour on him all the love she felt in her heart.

In each life, a veil on our consciousness prevents us from remembering why we make the choice of people, environments and experiences of that life. The mother in question, too, did not remember why her relationship with her son needed to be so arduous. She confessed to me that she would often lose patience while interacting with him, and get aggressive and sometimes even abusive when he exhibited aggressive behaviour. After her regression, she deeply understood that the complexity of their relationship intensified her need to practice patience, tolerance and unconditional love even under those trying circumstances.

In a stupor, after the session, slowly the mother was able to piece together the beauty of this powerful soul connection. In her review after two months, she expressed a lot of happiness over their improved relationship: no hitting, lots of patience and tolerance, and the fact that she was now able to exhibit her profound love for him. I asked her how much she thought she had changed, and she said, 'I have almost become a saint. My son is 50 per cent better.' Her husband also attested to this transformation in both the mother and the son. Even the child's IQ had improved by a few points. The transformation continued steadily, to the extent that her newfound patience had led her to start home-schooling her son!

I felt it imperative to explain to her that in addition to the karmic connection that her son had with her, he had his personal agenda and related issues to deal with in this life. It was, therefore, important that she should not expect that her personal transformation would trigger an equivalent response in him. Her child would not be able to change completely. With this awareness embedded in her, both of us settled into being curious and non-expectant observers of the child's developments.

In the last seven years, I have had five follow-up sessions with mother and son. Although a complete cure is difficult in autism, there have been changes in him that have significantly improved the quality of his life.

— —

These two cases of surrogate regression infused a lot of hope in me, especially as a parent and paediatrician. If we had not been able to establish this healing through surrogacy, we would have had to wait for a long time until the children were able to address them on their own. And it may have been too late by then, as their body may have lost its capacity to heal. I marvelled at the possibility of the changes that can occur through surrogacy, the solace that this understanding can bring to the anguished parents, and the renewed zeal that they could feel to help their child through many different complementary and supportive modalities.

More importantly, it taught me how sensitive physicians must be when disclosing any disturbing news to patients (in this case, the parents), especially mothers carrying babies in their wombs.

I hope that, with time, we will have enough scientific proof on integrated modalities of healing (regression, nutrition, movement therapy, and many more). So much so that competent doctors and therapists work hand in glove to nurture accepting yet proactive parents, and enable children to overcome their disabilities and experience a magnificent life.

In the light of this vision, it may be worthwhile to keep reminding ourselves that it all begins with that eternal, invisible connection—the cord of love.

In the Wake of Wisdom
Treating Multiple Syndromes Disorders in an Individual Through Regression

'It is a time when man and beast lived together in their glowing forms,' revealed my client during her session. This information about the past drew my attention to the present: today, we, as human beings, struggle to live in harmony with each other. Not only that, many of us find it difficult to be at peace with oneself. While the mind makes a quantum leap, the individual feels disintegrated in the physical, mental, emotional and spiritual spheres. During the time spent with my clients, I surprisingly discovered that the faculty of intelligence, which places humans at the pinnacle of evolution on Earth, is also capable of restricting the individual from further growth and refinement.

The healing journey of my client, Sindu, is intriguing in terms of its higher learning. While the other cases presented in this book mostly give us a clinical insight of regression therapy, Sindu's case awakens our vision to a broader perspective of this non-conventional form of healing, where my client delves into the realm of spiritual and higher wisdom. When awakened, such innate wisdom can shatter our own limitations and help us live a life of heightened awareness. This chapter is also exclusive in terms of its narrative: much of it is in Sindu's own words. It awakens us to the true potential of the *homo sapiens*, which literally means 'wise man'.

––

At forty-three, Sindu was the CEO of a publishing house with a fantastic international pedigree, accomplished and very well-articulated. She came with a history of multiple problems: obesity, chronic lower back pain and feet pain, rheumatoid arthritis, acute psoriasis, and Stevens-Johnson Syndrome—a rare and serious disorder of the skin in which the skin blisters and peels off.

Sindu's physical issues started manifesting for the first time in 1997, for which she took the aid of various orthodox and alternate medications, one after the other. She reported that while she made good progress with each treatment, her issues relapsed sooner or later. Being very well read, Sindu knew her situation was not terminal. Three years prior to approaching me, she had stopped all her medication since none of them had been able to give her a permanent solution. She said she had begun to sense there was something more to the physical manifestation of her issues.

As she recounted her history, I was able to gather an understanding of her traumatic and rebellious childhood and teenage years. Sindu had been an accomplished dancer even as a young girl, but had discontinued this art for which she seemed to have an unusual and inherent flair. She mentioned that she was obsessed with food and had gained a lot of weight around puberty. She ate whether she was hungry or not, and if her craving to eat was unsatisfied, it would result in a severe headache.

A few aspects of Sindu's personality became quite obvious to me over our first few interactions, and one of those was that there was definitely more than what was obvious. However, I did not foresee that, like an onion, there were several layers to her manifesting issues and healing would be synonymous with peeling all the layers to reach the core finally. My client admitted to feeling a severe void within and a self-defeatist attitude with time, but her outward projection was one of confidence and interest. Repeatedly, she expressed this idea of feeling like a fake and out of depth in almost all spheres of her life. While she felt happy to escape the control and authority of her home atmosphere when she moved abroad and enjoyed a successful professional life, she struggled to accept the new culture, internally. The unfamiliar environment made her feel quite weak, vulnerable and low on self-esteem. She continued to gain weight and suffered from other physical and psychological issues.

My interest in Sindu's case deepened as she recounted when her joint pain surfaced for the first time. She was visiting home on a holiday during her early twenties, and was thrown out of the house on her birthday when an argument blew out of proportions. As she narrated this incident, I could sense her pent up emotions: she was shocked and wounded that her own family was hurting her. Soon afterwards, she started suffering from acute pain in her joints and was diagnosed with rheumatoid arthritis.

The metaphor glared at me: rheumatoid arthritis is an autoimmune disease wherein the white blood corpuscles turn against the body; in other words, the body's immune system attacks itself. Intuitively, I was convinced that regression would certainly help Sindu; I felt she was ready for healing at all levels.

At the onset of her regression, Sindu mentioned that her weight bothered her the most. Until puberty, she was stick thin but started ballooning after that. However, even when thin and agile, she would look at her mirror, and was still not happy with her body and felt that she was not good looking. As she continued to gain weight, this feeling intensified. By the time she was in her forties, she was plagued with the feelings of being fat, ugly and a misfit in society. She felt judged and mocked at because of her weight, and bit by bit, she withdrew from people at large. It kept her from scaling professional heights and prevented her from enjoying the creative aspects of her life.

Food was an antidote all through. Eating helped her divert her mind from her inadequacies. If she didn't eat compulsively to meet emotional voids and disturbances, she would get migraine-like headaches. She had put herself into a catch-22 situation. The more mindlessly she ate, the more weight she gained. The more weight she gained, the more inadequate she felt, and the more she ate. She was sinking into the quicksand and was desperate for a lifeline. Interestingly, in the course of this exploration, she revealed that her ungainly and heavy body was not the only reason she hid from people. In her thirties, she developed a tendency to avoid people or situations as soon as she began to feel used or abandoned. Through her growing years, she had grown into a people pleaser, going out of her way to make people feel comfortable and help people. When her affection, time and energy was not returned, it not only stung, but she perceived it as a deep rejection and betrayal, quite an inflated reaction to a very normal and average experience of life.

When I probed deeper into the matter, she revealed that she overate whenever she felt unprotected, betrayed or threatened. Again, food was an antidote to her fears about people as she could avoid people, stay indoors, eat, and feel secure. Although she had mentioned earlier that food was an obsession for her, the fact that she ate to protect herself from others did not seem to make any sense to my rational mind. I found this piece of information quite strange: why would someone do that?

As she continued to ruminate about herself, she expressed fear. She was consumed by the fear that people would use her for her strengths, and deplete her energy, as she was a giver and not a taker. She was scared that she would have no one for herself when she needed someone. She was scared of being alone, suffering physically and then with a loud terrified sob, she exclaimed, 'I am scared that I will die a slow and torturous death. I will be alone; I will have no one to take care of me; I will die as a piece of rotting flesh.' And as she expressed this fear, she felt a tightness and pain in her legs, ankles, and toes.

It was time to take her back to the source of this fear of a horrifying death of rotting flesh. After making her comfortable with eyes closed and a few suggestions, I counted her back in time.

Me: As I count back from 5 to 0.
5. ... Move back in time to a situation where you are dying all alone and are scared.
4. ... Connect with the feeling when you are terrified that people around you are depleting you of your energy and strength and abandoning you, which devastates you.
3. ... Connect with the feeling of betrayal by people and the sinking feeling it has brought in you.
2. ... Intensify the inadequate feeling.
1. ... Move back in time to the lifetime when you feel more and more tightness in your stomach, ankles and toes.
0. ... Let the first impressions surface unnecessary. Describe what's happening.

Sindu: I am scared, as I am burning to death. There is fire all around me.

Me: How old are you?

Sindu: I'm a sixty-year-old male. Incapacitated, from my waist down.

Me: Look around you, what kind of a place are you in?

Sindu: I'm in a roomy home, a well-kept room. From a window, I can see lot of sheep and lambs around. There is a walking stick made of tree bark propped up against the wall. I'm lying on a square cot, have a long, white beard, a pale-yellow frock kind of a shirt and red pants.

Me: How badly are you incapacitated?

Sindu: I'm awake, unable to get up. I need help to stand as my legs are very weak ... She starts crying.

Sindu: My own children are doing this to me. Both my sons are watching me and not coming to rescue me. Nobody is helping me. How much I have helped so many people, so many people standing and watching me in the fire and yet no one ... (starts wailing).

Me: Look past the fire, at the people staring at you ... there are so many people ... do they all know you? Who are you to all of them?

Sindu: (In a very puffed up, proud voice): I'm Shamam, an Imam (worship leader), the chief of a tribal clan. I lost my wife when my children were very young. Along with my children, I raised the entire tribe. They all flock to me for my wisdom.

Sindu: The fire is touching me everywhere—arms, hands and feet.

Me: As you go through this painful experience, what else are you sensing in your physical body?

Sindu: There is something happening in my feet. I feel as if they are growing to a monstrous size ... they are not changing physically ... but I feel they have become like lead, heavy, as if my feet have become my body and my body has become my feet.

Me: What emotions are you going through?

Sindu: I don't mind dying. I am composed on the outside. But I am falling apart inside. I feel betrayed. There is a voice telling me to accept—let go ... but I am not listening to it; I am engrossed in this betrayal.

Me: Move forward towards the time of dying and describe what's happening.

Sindu: I am not feeling the pain. I am putting a lesson into my body—'Never go beyond and do anything for anybody, anyone. They will fail me'....

Me: What are your dying thoughts?

Sindu: I have closed my eyes, resigned ... I have an image of a young strong, able version of me, tough, not soft ... (spoken in a high-pitched voice with heavy, laboured breathing). The voice continues to ask me to drop the feeling of betrayal. I refuse....

She is breathing peacefully now. Although, she is describing her younger self, and while it would be logical to continue exploring the memory of the earlier part of her life that was surfacing, I decide to put it on hold and explore it a little later. My experience is that there is a lot of learning and wisdom that is arrived at during the moment of death, and hence the decision to pursue the time of death, first.

> Me: Look at your body, lying dead ... what do you observe?
>
> Soul: My body is burnt to ashes. I am calm, not anxious before dying.
>
> Soul: Wait ... I see all walking away, leaving me like that ... I'm surprised ... now confused.
>
> Me: Just connect with the people below to understand their behaviour towards you.
>
> Soul: What is it that made me suffer like this? What did I not learn? I was a very devout person; nobody is helping me; I am feeling unloved.
>
> Me: Keep going....
>
> Soul: As an Imam on Earth, I preached that if we do good, at the time of death, Allah comes to take us. There is no one to take me and I'm waiting....
>
> This is my moment of reckoning ... and in this moment, I am bottoming out. Beneath my piety, I see no faith. Beneath my wisdom, I see rigidity and beneath my gentleness, I see no compassion.
>
> Me: So, how does it connect with the fake feeling?

She had mentioned this feeling in her history session.

> Soul: I'm not just Shamam, but a total sham, a total fake....
>
> Me: And then what's happening?
>
> Soul: Ah ... Relief. I am surrounded by light. And as I soak into this light, this energy, understanding dawns ... I realise that I did not do what I was supposed to do. I led people the right way—but that was not enough. I led with power, not love. Most importantly, I deceived myself.

As Sindhu breathes peacefully, I let her relax and let this understanding sink in. I know that we have to travel back in this life to see where the deception started.

> Me: On my count—go back into the life of Shamam ... travel back to that moment where you will get a clear understanding of how it all started. What do you see?
>
> Sindu: A frame where I'm with my grandfather whom I adore. Both he and my father take care of the entire tribe. I'm five year old and my days are filled with hard work; I am devoted to helping with the sheep and the lambs and learning the scriptures, in preparation for the future.
>
> Me: Look at your grandfather; how do you feel in his presence and what kind of bond do you share with him?
>
> Sindu: He is my husband in my current life. The same energy of joy. It's like a stamp.

I see her reminiscing those happy childhood days. I let her enjoy it a bit and then move her forward to the next significant moment.

> Sindu: I'm sixteen years old. My father has died in an avalanche. My grandfather asks me to take the mantle of my father. Everything goes well—people ask me for direction, they bow to me, bring their children to me to name, and bless. Then a year later, my grandfather calls me and shares wisdom. He tells me, 'You are changing. You need to learn more, seek help and learn to listen. This arrogance can destroy you. Your ego is feeding you. I put the mantle on you too fast.' But, I pay no heed to it and laugh it away.
>
> Me: As I count you back from 5 down to 0, you will move to the next significant moment in your life. Describe what's happening?
>
> Sindu: I'm twenty-one years old, married with one child. My grandpa is growing very frail and soon he will die. A big part of me is also dying, big void, scared ... feel that when he dies, it will be like losing a backbone. Life continues ... no one to ground me.

I am solely responsible for healing, helping and I feel the stress and my legs are hurting.

Me: Connect deeper with your legs to understand, as to what are you storing in them.

Sindu: My grandfather has passed away. I don't have the depth and wisdom that all the previous Imams had. I'm quite shallow on the inside, not having spent time in deep reflection and understanding to develop myself. My inner voice keeps telling me, step down, contemplate, and spend some time in inner enquiry. However, the outer greed feeds my ego, glorification keeps me in the loop and I squash the inner voice. The web deepens and everything soon becomes superficial. My legs continue to hurt....

Sindu: My second son is born. I am unable to heal people; my prayers are not working. The glorious years of my ancestors are withering away in front of my eyes. My healing advice is going wrong. I am out of balance, no moderation. I hardly give time to my family. My legs are hurting badly.

Sindu: Two years after my second child, my wife passes on. Her loss is humungous—however, I push away all my feelings. The conflict continues between the inner voice of my heart and the outer glorification. My chest feels heavy. I enjoy the status, but feel fake and hollow. My legs feel heavy.

Me: Deepen the pain, the heaviness in your legs. Now, listen to the legs; what are they trying to tell?

Sindu: People don't know that I am fake. I don't have the courage to 'stand on my legs' and say that I am not the chosen one. Every time I face my cowardice, my feet hurt; this inability to stand up for the truth hurts me, hurts in my feet.

Me: As I count you back from 5 down to 0, you will move to the next significant moment in life and describe what's happening.

Sindu: Finally, things begin to dismantle. Fights sprout and as the discontent and divide deepens, I'm unable to bring the people together. My worst fears begin to take shape. My eldest son, Hameem, begins to expose me. In anguish, I go on a long walk.

The terrain is rocky and I trip over a boulder, hurt my lower back and tail bone, and become partially incapacitated from the waist downwards. My tribe asks me to allow Hameem to take charge. I agree, but stall, citing that he needs to train more. Oh my, I do not want to give it up. Hameem is doing well. I'm jealous and throw obstacles in his way. I'm creating a festering wound for my entire tribe and yet my ego refuses to sublimate.

Me: And how does it unfold in time?

Sindu: Ten years later, the festering wound has turned toxic and in its wake, I've been exposed completely. They decide it was time to remove the poison and cooperate to burn me alive. (Sindu starts crying and clamoouring after she says this statement.)

Through this long session of five hours, the yawning gap between the inner shallowness and the outwardly wise projections that deepened with time, surfaced. Throughout the recollection of this life, Sindu kept repeating, *'I am not able to stand up for myself.'*

This drew my attention to the fact that in the current life, Sindu suffered from chronic feet pain that prevented her from walking for long periods. As the regression progressed and she relived this hypocrisy, the excruciating pain in her legs began to surface.

Me: How does it feel to go through this experience?

Sindu: I helped so many of them and they let me down. They do not agree that I was of any benefit to them. If I help, I will be betrayed.

A part of her history flashed in me when I listened in on this. Even, in this life, she had a tendency to avoid people or situations as soon as she began to feel used, betrayed or abandoned. This feeling in her began to make sense now as she has carried over a strong sense of rejection, betrayal and self-pity.

I gently urged her to move forward in time, and when she reached a point where she was 'burning', I let Sindu relive the experience of being burnt in the fire, for I have found in my practice that a total release of psychosomatic conditions occurs only when the client is able to undergo complete catharsis. I guided her to breathe out all the memory of the fire, from every cell of her body and also release the ego, jealousy, hypocrisy from every pore and watch in what form it was leaving her body.

> Sindu: It leaves as a spiral of smoke, leaving from the lower half of my body. As it is leaving me, it is assuming the shape of Shamam.
>
> I'm confused. The image of when I got severely burnt with Steven John Syndrome is also coming up at the same time.

I decided to take this up for exploration after I completed exploring Shamam's life completely.

> Me: Relax, let's focus on Shamam....
>
> Me: Invite the five-year-old Shamam, and let him face the old Shamam. How does the old Shamam feel?
>
> Sindu: My training to become a leader was premature. My father chose to put me early in training at the age of five. I want to be a child first. The mantle feels too heavy and suffocating.
>
> Me: Good. Now move to when your father dies and when you took over. Are you ready to tear away that mantle and throw it away? Throw away the robotic unit that you are encased in?
>
> Sindu: Yes.
>
> Me: What do you see?
>
> Sindu: A black, heavy armour that's trapping me.
>
> Me: Look closely at it; are there any other impressions coming?
>
> Sindu: It belongs to the head priest of our tribe who died when I was very young. I have met him once. He was stabbed by my father's younger brother.
>
> Me: How do you recognise him?
>
> Sindu: His eyes, the fire in them ... the eyes are the same as my father's (current life father).

Sindu: The priest had also wanted to be glorified. He had also wanted to take my father's position.

Me: You knew all along that you were shallow and stepping down and stating the truth would have helped you to be well and contribute better in a more wholesome and guilt-free way. What stopped you?

Sindu: I could not.

Me: Please clarify.

Sindu: Because I was scared....

Me: Scared of what—that you will not have power?

Sindu: No.

Me: That people will not revere you?

Sindu: No (louder).

Me: That people will abandon you if they knew the truth?

Sindu: No (more loudly).

Me: Then why?

Sindu: (Screaming loudly) Because if I step down and stand on my two feet and tell them the truth, people will not give me the basic respect due to a human being.

I took a step back, a pause. What struck me really hard was that at the time of dying, Shamam had the feeling, *'At least treat me like a human being.'* As he was venerated as the head of a tribe, such a feeling seemed odd. I wondered about the sequence of lives that Sindu had gone through and knew that the pieces needed to fit together to see and understand this puzzle.

Sindu started developing connections between her past lives and current life instantly. While still in a state of trance, she questioned why she chose to live such a life of great deceit, not only to others around her but more so to her own self. My intrigue at her idea of 'fear of not being treated as a human' made me continue the session and she was very receptive.

I asked her to continue with her eyes closed and as I moved her back in time in the same life to when Shamam was struggling with the fear of his farce and his legs were slowly accumulating pain, she sought the reason for this fear. It took her back to life in the 16th century in which she saw herself as a well-built African tribal man, Ruka, with huge bulky legs.

Me: On my count from 5 to 0, go back to the first impression, the first fear of not being treated as a human being.

Sindu: I am feeling tremendous pressure in my legs … I am feeling the force of dichotomy … I am feeling fear in my legs.

Me: Continue, what is the first image you see?

Sindu: I see a bulky African man. He is bulky, muscular. Oh, wait it's me.

Me: How do you recognise?

Sindu: We have the same eyes.

Me: Continue.

Sindu: I have big, fat legs and my legs are in a heavy metal chain.

Me: What does the place look like?

Sindu: It's a cave-like structure made out of stone. I'm doing back-breaking labour work with the result that there are cuts across my body, which is glistening with sweat. My physical condition is precarious. However, on the outside, I seem very nonchalant. I have cloaked myself with a cold, brave and unaffected demeanour. I am a slave and it's obvious that I don't belong here. I've been brought from somewhere else. I'm building some kind of chamber; a secret chamber. I have a chisel and a hammer and a cutting device. I don't have any feelings in me. I'm numb. I don't let my body feel anything.

Me: How long do you work? How do you carry on?

Sindu: Water is stored in barrels and given to us in brown sheepskin sachets. We are also given only one meal a day made of burdock roots and charcoal-grilled meat.

As soon as she spoke about the food, her chest pained and she experienced laboured breathing. This was significant and I decided to explore it later. I acknowledged the pain, let her relax and moved her forward to the next significant moment.

> Sindu: I'm exhausted and I'm going to die. I have an open wound that is infected and I feel like I'm going into a state of shock. The soldiers dump me into a cave and close the opening with a boulder. I am alive in that dark cave with nothing; no food, water and left to die.
>
> Me: As you lie there, what are your feelings when you're ready to die?
>
> Sindu: I feel that I should have been treated like a human, at the least.

I moved her back to the time when the slavery started.

> Sindu: I'm about ten years old. I live in a village with my parents and brother. We are all dark-skinned and quite poor. Some soldiers come and pick us up and take us to a huge castle. The soldiers are light-skinned and we are presented to the Caliph (the king). He is wearing white robes with gold embossed all over it. He sits atop a throne and to reach it, one needs to climb a hundred stones. We are segregated. The women are taken separately.
>
> Me: What is it like with the men?
>
> Sindu: We get whipped constantly to continue working. The conditions of living are inhuman; one meal with some roots and meat. There is a lot of anger in me, especially over the food. I am hungry all the time; when served, I pounce on the food and shovel it down my throat like a glutton. The food I consume is not enough to feed this big body of mine and the stomach wants more and more. At the same time, my senses are in agony for losing control upon seeing this food and not resisting this one pithy meal served to me. The hunger is too overpowering. I slowly learn to control myself, and on the surface, I learn to pretend to the soldiers as if I don't care for this food. I suppress it and my chest is hurting.

It is the same chest pain she experienced when we began to explore this past life. The same emotion that produces disharmony between inner and outer feelings was occurring in this life, too— she feels (hunger) something inside and pretends something else (nonchalance) outside. My intuition tells me that this discord between the inside and outside will be a recurring theme through her regressions.

Me: Any inferences?

Sindu: My only companion in my part of the cave is another slave. He is more reconciled with the situation. However, I have disdain for his attitude and think of him as a weakling. As soon as the food is thrown at us, he is so grateful for the food and cries while eating it. His tears infuriate me, but no conversation is possible, as the soldiers would whip us. I glare at him all through our meals wondering why he can't swallow his sorrow and pretend to be brave like me … breathing quietly. Oh my, this companion of mine is my current-life mother.

Me: Where are you storing this anger in your body?

Sindu: My anger is consuming me. I bottled up all this anger, helplessness and restlessness in my legs that are continuously chained. What a terrible way to treat humans; even while defecating, we are chained. I feel trapped day after day and as my wound gets more and more infected, they push me into a cave to die a slow, rotten, stinking death.

I guide her to the time of death.

Sindu: This is such a terrible situation. Why me? What did I do to deserve such a life? Why can't people treat humans well? I'm intensely angry and so sad; my chest is paining. This life has treated me so unfairly with no ounce of comfort or tenderness. (Shallow breathing, as if going to die.)

Sindu (Making a resolution to herself): 'Never again will I be a slave. I will always be in the position of power, of authority. I will do anything to remain there, make any compromises. Never will

I bow to anybody, ever. I will always be in the position of power, of authority.'

This was an 'aha' moment for me. It would also become a moment of reckoning for Sindu, when she realised that it was this oath that shaped her next life—that of Shamam, the Imam. Usually, the thought one has, or the oath made by a person at the point of death determines their subsequent lives. This happens especially in the case of lives that are well-programmed when actually one is aware enough to contemplate the lifetime at the time of dying and there is time to plan the onward journey. The same is not the case with sudden deaths, like when one dies in an accident or out of a sudden terminal illness.

Even before I could commence the integration or prompt Sindu in that direction, she had begun speaking about how the life of Ruka had been a golden opportunity to experience and extend compassion.

> Sindu: This anger that I was trapped in was so destructive that I lost the learning of the whole life. I could have been compassionate and reassuring towards this companion of mine in the dark cave—the only human contact I had in this lifetime. Instead, I chose to be very angry and defiant. Had I used that opportunity to develop understanding, compassion and even empathy in me, I would have so much time and space to practice them and master all of these qualities.

She was in a very deep state and was reflecting on the lost chance to practise compassion. I prompted her to share her new wisdom.

> Sindu: If human beings, even in moments of abject adversity, rise and give from the core of their being, the source is never depleted. On the contrary, it is continuously repleted by the act of giving, which in turn is redeeming and uplifting for the being.

This statement was so profound and touching to me. I was lost for a moment in it. My intuition was telling me that this probably came from a very spiritual life of an evolved soul. I made a note of it and wondered what would unfold next.

During her resting time, Sindu shared that in her present life she had always felt as if she was her mother's mother, and could never react angrily over her mother's weaknesses. It was as if her wanting to capitalise on that lost opportunity of the past was ingrained so deeply that she deliberately chose to behave compassionately with her mother in the present. On the lighter side, my client revealed that she had *always* felt a stirring in her heart when she would watch her mother eat—a feeling that she had not been able to comprehend until that day!

As a part of the catharsis, I guided her to vent out her emotions and deep anger.

> Me: We can't change the events of Ruka's life. Pause and feel: if you are given an opportunity to let out all your pent-up wrath, what would you like to do?
>
> Sindu: I just want to break the chains and lash out at those guards and the Caliph.

I let her do it. I hold her legs with my hand, mimicking the chaining of her legs and ask her to break those iron bonds. This kind of body work helps release the associated stuck memories and provides better relief of physical symptoms. This release holds an important key to the ensuing healing. As she pushed against my hands and kicked free, she continued to envision herself escaping from the cave. I could see her breathing deeply and evenly and a feeling of relief began to come over her. Then I allowed her to release the memories of hunger by tapping her stomach. She mentioned that a sticky stuff was leaving her system and her stomach felt light.

> Me: You have experienced both the personalities from the past lives. There is in you now the wisdom that has come after releasing traumatic memories and emotions. Do you still want to hold on to all the negativity from Shamam's life?

Sindu: No, but I don't know if this anger will leave me ever. I wear it like a cloak around me.

Me: What is this anger? Where are you harbouring this anger?

Sindu: I have this anger and sadness at being used by people. I wear it like a cloak around me. I want to shake it off as I have met and befriended and had excellent relationships with some wonderful people. Yet I can't shake off this feeling.

Me: How do you want to release it?

Sindu: I want to tear it down and release it.

I place a thin pillow on her shoulders and tell her there is the cloak.

Sindu uses all the strength in her hands and pushes it away and sighs ... and feels as light as a feather.

I could have closed this session just having regressed her, facilitated catharsis and release. However, we were at a critical juncture to take the understanding and the wisdom gleaned and feed it back into her. I now took up the similarities between her current life and past two lives. I was astounded at the connection between these two lives, which made me understand that dealing with one part or aspect of the issue was not enough when another was already latched on to it. It was interesting to see how, in her present life, her feelings of being fake, her need to hide from people, her turning to food to deal with her own negative feelings of her body as well as fears of being betrayed by people, all emanated from these two lives of Shamam and Ruka.

As Ruka, she underwent abject humiliation and extreme hunger. She salivated over food, but her disgust for the slave owners, the soldiers and her own pride, made her project nonchalance on the outside. She left that body with a deep hunger for food, mastering fakeness (pretending to be unaffected by food on the outside), severe anger over being betrayed and used as a slave, and a soaring desire to always be in power and at the top of the chain.

So, she came into being as Shamam, at the top of the chain, continuing to use the mastery of hypocrisy to stay at the top, and died carrying the scar of rejection from her own people. In the present, the memory of the feelings of experiences in both these lives were triggered, one directly and the other, indirectly. Her relationship with her father, a taskmaster, directly triggered the memory of the feelings of the life of Ruka, evoking along with it the associated feelings of Shamam. The episode of Steven Johnson Syndrome experienced in this life directly triggered the memories of the feelings of the life of Shamam, making her retreat into her shell. It was amazing to see how these two past lives were interwoven and how they connected deeply with her current life. Even more fascinating was the realisation that the layers of the onion had already begun to peel off.

As Sindu relaxed after the regression, I gently guided her to reflect over the connections of her past lives with her current one. She was able to make the connections all by herself and began to speak immediately.

> Sindu: I have a dominant will power that is usually under my control. Strangely, when it came to disciplining my body, my will power failed always and there was only flight of desire and longing for a trimmer and more fit body. Whenever, it's time to work for myself (exercise, yoga, stretches, go to the beauty parlour, go for clothes or slippers shopping) I will just sit and eat. I don't want to push my body ... I will give some excuse or the other and avoid it. I'll procrastinate until I won't be able to do it later.
>
> I now understand my obsession with food. My father was a disciplinarian and a taskmaster. There was always so much to do (even as a child) and it had to be done well, else we would have to face the consequence of his anger. As a child, I felt terrified and suffocated with the need to work hard to please my father. In Ruka's life bogged down by hard work, there was no freedom and self-respect—the punishment was being treated as a slave with access to very little food. In this life, however, food was

freely available and it was easy to satiate myself with food to quell the rising feeling of fear, tiredness and of no freedom. The need to turn to food was programmed by its unavailability in Ruka's life, the memory of the life being triggered by my father's harsh demands. (Breathing quietly).

The next deep connection is that of the burning of Shamam and the horrific experience of suffering from Steven Johnson Syndrome in my current life. The sequence of events that happened in my current life are intriguing. My younger son was born with many food allergies and as I was nursing him, I gave up many, many food groups. A couple of months into this deprived eating rhythm, I began to shed weight copiously and was looking noticeably thin and smart. I remember relishing the shrinking jean sizes and enjoying my glowing skin and thinning appearance in the mirror.

However, on the inside, I was tired, drained and exhausted, keeping up a gruelling schedule of taking care of two children and nursing round the clock with a lower number of calories than required. I pretended to smile on the outside, but all the time, feeling gnawingly exhausted on the inside. I understand now that perhaps, the pretense, the hunger, being deprived of favourite food groups, intensified the memory of Ruka's life experiences.

One day, I looked at the mirror and the dichotomy was intensely staring back at me—of looking great on the outside and feeling like crap on the inside. The image was mocking me, 'This is how horrible it will feel inside in order to look so great on the outside'—the looming conflict between my inner and outer self.

Looking back now with my new understanding, this was the moment when the feelings of Shamam's life triggered. Within three weeks of this experience of staring at the mirror and a trigger of a feeling of being fake, internal heat began to spread through my body. There was an indescribable 'burning' feeling, my entire skin blistered (burnt) and peeled away, and facial features were completely distorted. I was overwhelmed and brought to my knees.

She was crying very softly, but with a deep understanding. I let her. Now that the catharsis, connections and understanding was crossed, it was time for integration, to seamlessly bring in the past lives into the current one and embrace the pain to erase it, another very critical step to healing.

> Me: Now, that you have understood the life of Shamam, gleaned all the mistakes made, released the cloak of hypocrisy and self-pity, are you ready to bring Shamam, free of all his problems into you? Look at him—he is outside of you, absolved of all that he carried. Are you ready to integrate him into you?
>
> Sindu: Yes, I'm ready.
>
> Me: Good. Allow Shamam to come inside you. Tell him that you understand the reason for the events, the hypocrisy, the rejection, the burning. You appreciate this Shamam, free of all his baggage. Welcome him.
>
> Me: How do you feel?
>
> Sindu: This healed Shamam is a part of me. I feel good, lighter, more at peace. I understand so much more....

Sometimes integration is not this beautiful. The person will resist, be fearful, feel awkwardness or experience downright discomfort. In such cases, the therapist understands that the work is incomplete. There are emotional threads (same life or linked to a different life) that are unresolved and need to be explored.

Although the first session had been quite intense, I felt as if I could have completed all her sessions in one whole day if it had been so possible to accommodate them in my schedule, because of the connecting thread that ran through her lifetimes. But I had to push the pause button, mainly so that it would give her the time to digest and assimilate all that she was beginning to learn and unlearn. The gaps between the sessions were also crucial for the healing to manifest at all levels.

--

During her first review, Sindu shared the very encouraging news of her healing. The first big change that she had moved into was a reduction in her emotional eating. She exclaimed that she did not have to exert her will to do it, rather it happened quite naturally and spontaneously. In the last session, we had gone over two past lives and peeled two layers of the onion. In the first life regressed (one layer) she arrived at the sequence of events that led to intense feelings of betrayal, rejection, self-pity and fatal dismissal. In the second, she relived intense hunger and situations that deeply affected her self-respect and how food was a panacea for her emotional issues in this life. By peeling this first layer, multiple issues were peeled off.

I decided to give a gap so that she could live her new learning before our next meeting. But when I saw her exactly four months later, her weight had increased by four kilograms. She said that while she liked to exercise, persisting joint pain prevented her from doing so. Also, her skin seemed to be bothering her more now; she had suffered from another attack of psoriasis during the course of time.

Through the months that followed, Sindu regressed through a number of lifetimes and integrated the lessons from each one of them in a similar fashion. We addressed her joint pain and skin problem, which again called for multiple layers of healing that was connected to more than one past life. Each lifetime that she went through opened easily and connected with every facet of her current life.

Whether it was the life of the Chinese prostitute where she was used mainly for her beauty and her body, or the life of Kian in ancient India where he went through deep and rigorous spiritual training but ended up becoming a renegade, or the life of an extremely beautiful Indian woman, married to a fisherman and dying all alone prematurely due to abuse and neglect, or the life of Maria, an African woman in 18th century Libya, who marries for love, is tortured by her father-in-law, loses her husband in an accident, delivers a still-born child and sets herself on fire, exhausted, and unable to continue living, the running thread of emotion through all her lives was the fear of being used and thrown away. This suppressed emotion from the past was ruling her present to the extent that it had adversely affected her holistic sense of well-being.

I could make out how much Sindu had been storing in the current life, especially as a child. She had been emotionally burdened, rather bloated up with emotions, if I may say so. It was, therefore, important to address every traumatic memory that she had carried since childhood and let go of these emotions that were built up at different ages, in different situations and with different relationships. With every layer that she let go, she got better, and this is how she narrates her healing experience:

'The first thing I found was that I was beginning to accept myself for who I am. As I experienced and understood all that my body had been through in so many lives, it was easier to accept and forgive. It was as if the mind was sending signals to and receiving signals from the body. This experience reinforced the idea—always believe in: that the mind and body have to work together to heal. Soon, I began to stand up for myself. I learnt to say "No" where needed and draw a line to protect my own space. I also started feeling less dependent on other people, and I was not so volatile in my emotions. So, there was a lot of change, though it may not have looked so apparent from the outside. But I could feel it and that's very important. I was even able to cope quite well with the fear of failure and rejection.

'At the physical level, my joint pain reduced and I was able to walk very well. The pricking sensation that I had in my feet all the time, which prevented me from walking, went away. I would not say I lost weight, but I was definitely not gaining weight. My tailbone and lower back pain got better. After the session in which we addressed my skin problem, the psoriasis and eczema that I had been long suffering from, completely healed. Additionally, in between lives during that regression, I gained the knowledge that my body had a mechanism to remind me of my higher purpose. So, every time I did something that went against the grain of what I believed in, my skin would start itching, showing me that I was going wrong. When I saw the therapist again after eight months, I was a lot better but I still had a little pain in my joints that restricted me from exercising and dancing.'

I was very curious to know what stood in the way of her using her body as she did seem to project a fine will power. Sindhu is extraordinarily passionate about dancing. Whenever she spoke about dance, her eyes would sparkle. She shared that she started classical dancing at the age of five, gravitating towards a teacher all by herself, and moved into deeper and more arduous dances very quickly. I was fascinated at hearing her describe her performances. She started stage performances very early and by the age of twelve was performing three-hour-long individual shows.

She said that when dancing, she was in a different world, completely yoked to the Divine. Everybody melted away; it was just her and the Divine, nobody else. She danced in that space and was very unaware of crowds, adulations and the glory that followed. She gave up dancing of her own accord around the age of sixteen when she realised the corruption and commercialisation associated with it.

The greed and manipulation of her teachers and community towards performances and achievements was heart-breaking and she broke clean from it. However, dance still remains her chosen form of exercise over any other. Therefore, the block she felt towards dancing even to exercise or experience happiness was puzzling to me. She kept assuring me that her weight and the pain in her joints prevented her from dancing.

I was not convinced, however. You see, her body and spirit seem to be speaking something else and this observation was very pivotal for me. From the first day, I had observed that joy and happiness were missing in her. I had a clue: the fact that she had closed her doors to dance, the one form of activity that gave her immense pleasure, had robbed her of all joy and happiness. Her withdrawal from dance was for reasons more than those purely physical. We decided to explore what the block was and a most fascinating session unfolded that took her back to a time before civilisation where all beings lived in harmony with Nature and with each other.

--

Sindu's life as Tiara, a healer, was one of purity and beauty of the heart. It opened my vision to the wisdom of our ancients and the oneness of Creation. Sindu's regression to this lifetime was fascinating. During this session, the energy in my own clinic seemed different as Sindu began to share, reciting all of this in an almost poetic form.

After making her comfortable and letting her focus on her breathing, I began to count her back in time.

> Me: At 5 … You are moving back in time to another life, another place where you were a good dancer … but something went wrong….
> 4 … Let your mind be open and connect with a happy memory of that lifetime where you are so passionate about dancing….
> 3 … As the impressions surface, connect with that experience deeply….
> 2 … What kind of place is it? Who are you? How does it feel being there?
> 1 … Let first impressions surface….
> 0 … Whenever you are ready, please describe what you see.
>
> Sindu: It is a time, even before civilisation, when man and beast lived together in their glowing forms. There is spectral light all over the Earth. Even in the darkness, after sunset, there is luminosity, and all creatures seem to be glowing with it. The living forms are not solid at all, and although I can feel the body, it is very light. All the animals seem very mystical, and there are even some tiny luminous beings that seem to move from flower

to flower without their feet touching the ground. The flowers are of exotic colours, with their own rhythm of opening and closing.

Me: Can you see yourself? Who are you?

Sindu: I am a healer, like the shamans. We heal through music, dance and movement. Through such movement, we enter an altered consciousness, and acquire wisdom and ability to heal people holistically. All creatures, including the flowers, bees and butterflies, open in rhythmic movement, and absorb the messages of healing. The person who is not at ease, who is in disease, is brought into the circle of dance, and the healer in this state of altered consciousness enables healing. There is so much of joy in this healing process, even for the diseased person. It is so graceful and harmonious as if all of Creation is one. Everybody, without exception, even people who are well, participate in this ritual-dance, because it is their way of connecting with the Higher Spirit.

I lead, singing and dancing so many times. (It's fascinating, there is no tiredness). As I perform the healing song and dance, so much of love and energy flows into me and from me to whoever is around. This is healing energy. I feel like an angel walking on Earth. It is pure ecstasy.

There are no houses—in fact, there are no indoors. But when we need an isolated place with some privacy, for example, at the time of mating or giving birth or feeding the child, we bend two long trees (that look like bamboo) towards each other, knot them firmly together at the top and hang all sorts of creepers on them to form a canopy-like structure. In case of marriage and union, we hang creepers with cordate leaves, which are heart-shaped, over the two sticks that we tie together. When somebody passes on, we don't bury the body; instead we leave it under the same structure covered by leaves that resemble a boat to suggest the pass-over. The body is left to rot naturally under the canopy, and in three days, the ritual is over. When a mother is going to deliver, we use leaves that have a spindle on the top, but a broad red base symbolising the baby coming out of the mother's body in a natural way. The mother delivers the baby all by herself, and only after the baby is heard crying, does someone go in to assist her.

We don't do things just because we have to do them, and we exhibit so much of beauty, grace and innate wisdom when we put these structures together. Our 'house' is very natural and can be easily dismantled; so when the ritual is over, we just release the trees back without causing them any harm. We don't seem to cook—I don't see any fire at all—but we know exactly which fruits, roots, seeds and nuts are meant to be eaten. And if somebody gets hurt, we squeeze these leaves on the wound and the skin comes back immediately. We bathe in the rivers, and we are required to maintain certain postures with our bodies to keep them fit. We have absolutely supple bodies, and one can hardly make out any wrinkles.

We know what to use, what not to use, and although it all seems magical, it is not magic. These wonderful people spend their days and nights in rituals dedicated to building their body and their spirit. And not everybody can be a healer; you have to be born as one.

Me: How is a healer identified?

Sindu: At birth, there is a glow around the child; so they know that a healer is born. These healers are highly intuitive: they reside in a space in their hearts from where the Earth is very transparent to them. They don't use their mind so much like the way we do now. So, the wisdom, the spirit with which they conduct themselves, their integrity and their ability to hold the whole clan up above are the determining qualities of the one who continues to be a healer.

Me: So, you are a healer ... What else is happening in this life? Other than the ritual dances. Do you have a family?

Sindu: There is another wonderful dancer I am drawn towards. His energy attracts me and he is a very important being for me. (Oh, that's my husband in this life—same eyes). All joy is short-lived. There are people who will not let me be with him.

Me: Who are these people?

Sindu: There is a man with a long beard and bushy eyebrows. His eyes are sharp and piercing and when he sees me, there is an energy that is dark that pierces into me. (Oh, that's my father in this current life—again). This energy is so strange and foreign to this beautiful, pristine place we live in. This man is the chief of the whole tribe. Why does he not like me? Why is there a mismatch in energy?

Me: Move forward, what happens then?

Sindu: They do not allow me to be with him as he is not a healer. There is a strange imposition in this almost magical land. Healers are allowed to unite only with healers. No one is ready to help me. My beloved is unable to do anything. Both of us are helpless. The chief announces the marriage of his daughter to my beloved and I am to perform the wedding ritual songs and dance.

Me: How do you feel?

Sindu: I am broken. I am turning dark, no joy. How to perform? I am experiencing a new emotion though. I am scared of the chief. I'm in despair. What is the point of being a healer? What is the point of being such a fine dancer? Dancing and healing did not get me what I wanted the most. I feel anger (with the chief's father for making such a rule), sorrow (that my mother is not with me), guilt (did not listen to my father), hopelessness (for my future), and frustration (cannot express my sadness as I must dance and sing with joy). I showcase happiness. My performance is brilliant because I am consuming myself and performing.

Me: Move forward to the next significant moment ... what happens?

Sindu: I have performed at my beloved's wedding. All of my vital energies have left me. I am lying on the ground turning dark. I take a resolution not to dance anymore. My body feels gross; every cell of my body is hurting. No one is around me. And as I leave my body, my two main thoughts are:

    I WILL NEVER DANCE AGAIN
    I WILL NEVER HEAL AGAIN

    I feel the essence of these oaths percolating into every cell.

I let her feel this oath, take her through dying and then the wisdom....

> Soul: As I see my body, I feel as if my body has failed me. If I had not been a dancer, healer, I would have been permitted to be with my beloved. I'm also perplexed. There is no dark side in life by itself. It is these man-made laws that make it dark.

She continues to be suspended in that state where she is processing the meaning of this life and then exclaims….

> Soul: This lifetime was pristine and one of proximity to nature. But since I had never been exposed to any impurity or negativity until I was eighteen, I didn't have the mechanism to adapt to change and accept the suffering that came with losing the love of my life to someone else. I chose to perish rather than live without love; all the light and joy was sucked out of my being and I was wrapped by the darkness of negativity. Now, I realise that how much ever we open and connect to the Creator, if we are not willing to let go of our dark side, it can darken us completely.

A few weeks after this particular session, she shared her understanding. 'As I learnt the reason that held me back from dancing, I was able to completely get rid of the joint pain, overcome my inhibitions, and bring this joyful and inspiring art back into my life, slowly but surely.

'I also understood that it was not the nature of the medicines I took earlier that caused the relapse, but it was actually the presentation of the "trigger", which was nothing but one or more of these emotions that I had for long-suppressed within myself. When I look back at the sequence of events, I feel all the treatments were successful but they could not get past any trigger. It has been more than a year and none of the issues that were dealt with during regression have relapsed. I now feel motivated enough to pursue what I have missed the most in life. There is also an opening, a sense of freedom from within, which makes me feel safe to pursue my dreams.'

Clearly, along with healing of the mind and body, Sindu had grown at a deeper level and I was amazed at the wisdom she now seemed to possess. However, unlike the past, her wisdom was not faked but was integrated with her very being.

My sessions with this very receptive client were revealing to me in more ways than one. They not only taught me to be very alert to every single statement that a client spoke during regression, but they also drew my attention to the paramount significance of listening to the heart. When we are in our heart, there is no hypocrisy: the inside and the outside are the same. Whenever the mind intervenes, if we are able to shut its chatter and turn our attention to the voice of the heart, we would have made the most of the opportunity or situation we are presented with at any given point in time.

About four months later, our review session showed much better progress on all fronts, except this hypocrisy, this feeling of inside-outside being different that still haunted her. In the ensuing session, we regressed to the setting of a life in Europe long before Christ was born.

> Sindu: I am an extremely rich, mean and ruthless moneylender. I'm Noel, about sixty-year-old male, Jew, stout, wearing clothes that exude prosperity.
>
> Me: What else do you see?
>
> Sindu: A lady who borrowed money from me. She is dressed in a white shirt with a blue skirt, tightly coiled hair. She seems like she'd be thirty years old and has an eleven-year-old with her. (Oh my, that's my son in this life). It's the market place. I am slightly drunk and on a high that I am the only one with money. All the others do barter trade. I have an assistant who keeps a long paper of accounts and the lady is begging me to give her some more time.
>
> Me: How are you reacting?
>
> Sindu: I tell my assistant to get the boy, drag him through the market and take him as a slave. The mother is crying, begging and pleading. There is so much of wisdom, fearlessness and courage radiating from the little boy's eyes. I can't bear those eyes as I feel

they are penetrating the depth of my consciousness. In anger, I set fire to him and burn him and there is a smile on my face. As the boy dies, he is not perturbed; he does not beg and scream for help. As my eyes meet the eyes of the boy perishing, my inebriated state leaves me and his eyes bore into me.

Me: How are you feeling?

Sindu: His eyes do something to me. They tug and pull at the deepest part of my heart. But, I'm too arrogant and proud. I mask it, then ignore it. The next day the mother confronts me, crying and shouting and telling people that this is the price she paid for borrowing money from a barbarian. As I watch her cry, again there is a pull in my heart and a churning in me. There is so much love in her eyes for her son. I am envious that I have not experienced that kind of love. She pines for her son (Oh wait, she is my daughter from my current life).

My legs are hurting….

Me: What does this feeling do to you?

Sindu: I begin to feel very tired and soon the situation and feelings are changing. I am pining as to why my money can't buy me love. Gradually, I'm losing my shrewdness. People cheat me. (Begins to cry softly.)

Me: As I count from 3 to 0, you will move to the next significant moment and get impressions….

Sindu: I'm about seventy years old. People are stoning me to death in the marketplace (crying loudly). I see the form of that mother and son, the son whom I burnt. I ask, 'Have you come to mock me?' She says, radiating a glowing love, 'We are all one. I will come again in some other life and give you the love you need. Do not worry, we are all connected.'

I let her cry and guide her to the moment of death.

Me: How do you feel? What are your thoughts?

Sindu: As I die, I think will they forgive me?

Me: As a soul, how do you feel looking at your whole life?

Soul: I feel sorry that I wasted my whole life.

Me: What makes you feel so?

Soul: I could've done so much good. I let the power of money just go to my head. I made a lot of mistakes. I had so many chances to be fair, just and kind and still retain my wealth.

I let her assimilate these lessons and decided to take her back to this lifetime to see what events had transpired to make her into this kind of a jaded person. I give a simple suggestion to move to that point of time to understand where she assimilated that behaviour.

Sindu: I lived in a beautiful house made of cobblestone. I live alone with three male servants to take care of me. It's all about money for me.

Me: What changed you into a ruthless money-minded man? Go back in time when it started.

Sindu: I am a five years old. It's the fasting season for Jews. We have a harmonious family. I'm very fond of my mother (Oh, it's my husband in my current life) who has a radiant beauty. Our house is a rectangular structure; many such houses make up a block. We are hardworking, loving, and devout, read the scriptures every day and abide by the Torah. The whole community is beautiful.

I let her enjoy the experience. And then take her to the next significant moment.

Sindu: I am about twelve years old. The land belongs to a rich Jew. He is obsessed with my mother and wants to claim her. On a Sabbath day, he sets fire to our home, rapes my mother and throws her into the raging fire (starts to howl and cry). I am witness to all this as I had escaped and was hiding in the bushes.

Me: How are you feeling and what thoughts are crossing your mind?

Sindu: My blood is boiling and I vow in silent fervour to take revenge. I go to the Jew, fake total helplessness and plead and beg to be employed by him. I work hard for him to trust me; I press his feet, bring him his food, drinks and cater to his every small need. With every passing day, he trusts me totally and I bide my time. He's a man without a conscience, consumed totally by money and power. One night, when he is completely drunk, I stab him with a dagger, take all his money, and ride away with two of his horses. The terror in his eyes at the time of death gives me the satisfaction of having avenged my parent's murder.

I let the feeling wash over.

Me: Proceed … where do you go next?

Sindu: I reach a poor but bustling place. A sharp sense tells me that if I play my cards right, I can be the richest man here. By now, the idea that money is everything, that money holds power is ingrained in me. I decide to forget my past and move forward. If my family was rich and powerful, bad things wouldn't have happened to us. I want to be rich and powerful. I bury the money in a safe place.

Me: And then what happens? You are still young; how did you move forward…?

Sindu: I meet a wonderful Rabbi (Jewish priest) in the market (Oh, he is one of my professors in college whom I was quite fond of). He is very popular and I ask him for protection. He takes me under his wing, nourishes, nurtures and moulds me. Despite being shown the right way by him and seeing him live the scriptures every day, I couldn't shake off the deep desire to be rich and powerful.

Me: And then, what happens?

Sindu: When I am seventeen years old, the Rabbi dies. He had so much of hope that I would continue his lineage of service. However, I have different plans. I take out all the money that I hid and the money he had marked for service and begin to lend.

Me: What does the money look like?

Sindu: Silver and copper coins. There are some symbols on them that I don't recognise. I'm a very shrewd and successful lender. People trust me as I have been held and showcased by the benevolent Rabbi. With time, the ruthlessness within me surfaces. I want people to experience pain the same way that I have experienced it. Soon, I don't know how to live without this money; I get people to beg and plead with me for mercy.

Me: Go forward. How long does this go on?

Sindu: After a while, I begin to tire. The same conflict arises. My inner voice tells me that I'm not enjoying this. It is directly in conflict with whatever the Rabbi and my parents stood for. But, my mind feels pleasure. (She's connecting dots in her mind in this trance itself and exclaims, 'It is that same dichotomy again.')

I move her forward to the end of her life and allow her to look back.

Me: What are your lessons?

Soul: The mantle of being a rich man and being warped in the pleasure of money lets me move away from my inner voice. I failed myself in being one integrated person, yet again.

Me: Do you still need to hold onto the mantle? What do you want to do with it?

Sindu: I want to drop it and I realise that I was holding onto it. Now, I don't have to ... it's just melting away giving me huge relief, with a feeling of gentleness sinking in....

As the grossness of power melted away from her, I brought in front of her, the five-year-old Noel.

Me: Standing before you is the innocent five-year-old Noel, before the twisted turn of events. It's Noel who has not witnessed the massacre of his parents. Look at his innocent eyes and connect with him. Tell him that all the anguish is over. He is safe to relive and experience his innocence, gentleness and tenderness.

Sindu: Yes ...

Me: Are you ready to integrate this five-year-old Noel?

Sindu: Yes.

Me: Invite him in, give him a big hug ... How does it feel?

Sindu: It feels nice. The arrogant person that I grew into in that life, the memory of which I carried in my current life is not me anymore. This innocent, gentle person feels like me.

As a paediatrician, this particular session of Sindu's was important for me. It reaffirmed my belief that a little twist in the life of a young, innocent child, colours them so much, that they take on the very twist as their identity. It is very important that children go through safe childhoods (not pampered, luxurious and indulgent ones), but where they are emotionally safe and have love-filled childhoods. This provides them with a strong base that allows them not to be corrupted as the years fill out and face what comes with stoicism and poise.

By the end of September 2018, Sindu had made considerable progress. Through each regression, she had peeled layer after layer to heal from complex problems. First, she peeled off hypocrisy, betrayal and the burning of her skin. This helped her work on her feelings of inner and outer discord, leg and joint pains and feeling used and abandoned by her friends and acquaintances. In the next layer that she peeled, she came to terms with her life as a slave and the issues of emotional eating. To her delight, she was able to overcome her mindless eating. The next layers that got peeled helped her diminish her inner and outer disharmony. The next layer that got peeled helped her with her psoriasis. Her deep love for dance as a divine art but being unable to practise it, was resolved with the next layer that peeled.

As we proceeded in this way, with the integrations, her reflections, her alertness to repeating patterns and the need to use her will power to let go and be true to the new person that she had now become. She began to feel more whole, exuded vitality and was filled with the confidence that she could live a new life.

Sindu's regression sessions also included interactions with her spirit guides in between two lifetimes. These 'rest' periods were laced with deep insight and understanding of why she had chosen her present life as it was.

The first happened after she had regressed to experience the extremely difficult, painful and lonely life of a beautiful fisherwoman, battered and abused by a violent, drunk husband.

> Soul: I'm going to a place of rest, a dimension in which I will have time to reflect and introspect. I'm not filled with light. The energy is a mixture of darkness and light. My guide (an illuminated energy) presents itself to me and asks me to rest as much as I want.
>
> Soul: I feel restless as I have to figure out a way to practise forgiveness for this violently abusive husband of mine. I don't want to reincarnate and not forgive.
>
> Guide: There is eternity to practise. To do it right away is your choice.
>
> Soul: Another energy joins my guide in this conversation. It is the same person who had been very kind and gentle to me in the difficult life that I had just relived. He says he is ready to come down with me to help me practise forgiveness. He chooses to come with me as my spouse. I now have to choose in incarnating with the violently abusive husband of that past life as either my sibling, son or father.
>
> Guide: You may choose the role of father. You will have extended time and a spectrum of situations to practice forgiveness. One life is not sufficient to master such deep vibrations. It will be better to choose him as father.
>
> Soul: The resonance is immediate and I choose to incarnate with him as my father.

The next interlude in which she interacts with her Guide to choose her next incarnation is fascinating. It happened after the life of Kian, a person who was bestowed with enormous amount of wisdom and knowledge and became a rogue renegade at the end.

Soul: My guide and I discuss the intent of the life that had passed. I had chosen that life with all its tests so I would not succumb and would strengthen values. However, I repeatedly succumbed. We go over all my mistakes, each incident, what I could have done differently, the choices that I was primed for, yet had deviated from. It's now time to choose the next incarnation.

Soul: I will go again, but this time I don't want any of the power, glory and fanfare. I want all of the learnings packed into one life. I WILL learn.

Guide: It's going to be difficult. Perhaps, it would be easier to break all of the lessons into smaller capsules to experience and learn from many lives.

Guide: You may choose a life where you are aware of your choices and yet you choose to achieve and succeed with all the right values. This would be the first step in a series of learnings.

Soul: No, I've wasted many lives. I want to accelerate. I accept the challenges and difficulty.

Guide: Let's look at your spectrum of choices of lives.

Soul: I choose the toughest life.

Guide: At every turn, you will be aware of your potential and capabilities. Two ways to manifest them will be available: the easy way, fully absorbed in yourself and the enormously difficult, yet correct way that will cultivate humility, compassion, vision, quietness, benevolent leadership and an alignment with the higher purpose.

Guide: This will be very tough. The option is still available. You can still choose to split all of this learning across lives, if not in a life after life sequence, at least across many lives being lived at the same time.

Soul: I am determined to learn and practice. I stay with my choice of choosing one tough life.

Sindu: My guide doesn't interfere with the final choice. A guide's role is only to suggest.

These two interludes were pivotal for Sindu. She realised how she had chosen every suffering for her own evolution. She, therefore, began to appreciate and be grateful for her pain. Everything that seemed negative and terrible as a child, began to feel purposeful. She no longer led an unaware life—her awareness had heightened—and in the wake of this wisdom and realisation, she was working with her will to make herself better.

One of the issues that stuck out as a sore thumb, even after many sessions spanning over three years, were her unresolved feelings for her father. On the one hand, she was afraid of him and also angry with him and on the other hand, in a completely opposite emotion, she felt the pull of the same flesh and blood and was always running to run errands for him and to please him. During her history-taking session, she shared her diagnosis of rheumatoid arthritis (RA), an autoimmune disorder in which one's own body turns against itself. The metaphor now glared at me. She perceived her father, her very own, to be not on her side, as someone who was attacking her all the time.

Over the span of various lifetimes that we regressed into, we found that in all, she and her father had been at crossroads in very violent and humiliating ways. I could see that she was struggling to forgive him yet was unable to be compassionate towards him. In one session, to understand why she was inviting the same soul again and again in the same equation, he as the perpetrator and she as the victim, and suffering, I gave her a suggestion to move back into her lifetime where she may have been the perpetrator.

As usual, she was very receptive to the suggestion and found herself in a lifetime where she was a male official in the court of a King and is locked in an aggressive battle with another colleague for a very high-ranking position. That colleague was her father in her current life. To reach that powerful position that held glory of power, wealth and fame, she plotted to kill her colleague. She created a fire accident and burned him to death. While dying, there is burning rage and hatred in her colleague's eyes. He curses her and tells her that he would never forgive what she had done to him and that he would exact his revenge.

Thus rid of him, she enjoyed the power, position, and wealth, that the undisputed appointment brought her. Her consciousness was so base and replete with greed that she had no remorse for what she had done till she died in that life.

At the end of this very short regression, she stayed quiet, stunned by this revelation of a life in which she had been the perpetrator. The understanding also dawned on her that this one unjust life of greed, mercilessness and cruelty had invited such a deep hatred and wrath from her colleague that life afterlife, she had to play out the victim to pay her dues, as her colleague extracted his pound of flesh. This vicious cycle of the roles of the victim and the perpetrator, depending on the experiences and oaths taken, gave her a deep understanding of the nature of her relationship with her father.

Very flippantly, we use the phrase in India: 'It is all my karma.' Little do we realise how profoundly true this is. Sindu experienced it through the roles she played. She was hungry for this wisdom and embraced it gratefully. She resolved to let go and change her reaction patterns with her father, using this understanding as the foundation. In the first few months after this regression, she said that though it was difficult, she generously practised it and it did give her great relief from this heavy burden on a daily basis. Her practice of meditation and letting go helped immensely in deepening the wisdom that she acquired from the session.

Over a period of a year and a half, she shared that the way she had assimilated this understanding and wisdom within her had changed her way of thinking. The reaction process was fantastic. 'Every time I am with my father now, I see the foundation (the understanding that I have also played the role of the perpetrator) and this precedes my interaction with him. Thus, although he is his usual self, the glasses through which I see him, hear him, observe him, and understand him is now different. My reaction is, therefore, also different. Most times, I have actually experienced compassion for him. And there is perhaps a very quiet part inside me that deeply apologises for my greed and the hurt I inflicted on him. This is a huge change: from being hurt by him, by discrediting him, I have moved to compassion for him.

'Who knows this wisdom may cleanse me so much and make way for the real love (which I do feel I have for him deep within) to come out and be expressed. I also have come to appreciate how wonderful this awakening is. I am no longer living in illusion any more. I know that sometimes, despite the foundation being awakened, when the situation gets uncomfortable or aggressive, that understanding refuses to surface. In such cases, I am able to very naturally ignore and put distance, without creating a baggage of frustration, sadness or anger. In all, a remarkable transformation—all by this snippet of a regression that gave way for a keen and beautiful understanding.'

In February 2020, I received a call from Sindu, eighteen months past her last session. She said that she was not doing well. Her blood work was still normal and stable (RF negative, normal CRP/ESR). She had no joint swelling or any other symptom of rheumatoid arthritis, other than severe joint pains. But, more than anything, she was in anguish as her body had not shed even one kilogram of weight. I first did a history session of the past eighteen months. Normally, the first success in weight loss is stopping the weight gain and then remaining static as fat is lost but muscle mass increases; but in her case, it was surprising that she was not losing weight, since the response to therapy is usually evident in six months. As I explored further, I realised that she was in a complete hate relationship with her body. She felt swollen; every time she made an effort to lose weight, she felt like she had to torture her body to look even decently good. She felt ugly most of the time, imbalanced, disgusted with herself and, above all, embarrassed by her body too. It was all about the body.

There was a striking analogy that she used. She said, '*I feel that the sheath of energy around me is always disturbed. It is like a bloated balloon. It can never settle down. The only way to smoothen it is by torturing myself with exercise and yet I do not get results. I go through hell, will look good for a bit and then fall sick and crash completely.*'

I was very curious about this sheath of energy that was bloated, and using the above statement as a bridge, I regressed her to the life of Mary, an Englishwoman in the sixteenth century.

> Me: (After a brief focus on her breathing and calming her down, I guided her to move back as I count down from 5.)
> 5 ... Move to the lifetime where you harboured the feeling of hatred of your own body.
> 4 ... Connect deeper with the feeling of the disturbed sheath of energy around you.
> 3 ... Let your mind open up to the memories where your body underwent torture.
> 2 ... Allow the memories of that lifetime to surface, where your relationship with your body is one of disgust, embarrassment, imbalance and swelling of your body.
> 1 ... Deepen the feeling, where you decided to live out of your body.
> 0 ... And what do you see, first impression, first image, first scene.
>
> Sindu: I am a seventeen-year-old, beautiful and elegant orphan. I live in the same orphanage that I was raised in. People here are gentle and kind. It's my home. I am very well-read and I teach the children of the orphanage. By disposition, I am positive, don't grudge my situation or have any self-pity. I try to do as many odd jobs as possible to bring money into the orphanage for our needs. I'm a beautiful (Wow!) and cheerful person.
>
> Me: Move to the next significant moment in that lifetime to understand more about that life.

Sindu: A sixty-year-old man is totally besotted and wants to marry me. The thought is a little revolting as he is the age of a parent to me. I still agree to the proposal.

Me: Why are you agreeing?

Sindu: It's obvious. It's a time-old trade. He pays money to have me and I agree out of gratitude to the orphanage and hope that they will have a better life. The glitter of hope and expectation in the eyes of the children helped me make the decision in a heartbeat.

Me: How is life feeling after the wedding?

Sindu: I'm a trophy wife. I don't have the right to feelings. I wear the best clothes, live in a mansion, and have everything that money can buy. I am numb though. He treats me well for all those who can see.

Me: What does that mean?

Sindu: I thought he bought me to be a trophy wife and to give him pleasure. I was totally wrong. Pleasure, yes, however, totally twisted pleasure. He is a revoltingly disgusting man. He has a manservant with him all the time. A horrendously scary looking man. Whenever, my husband is angry with me or wants to assert his conjugal rights on me, he lets him on me, to take me, rape me.

Me: What does your husband do? Where is he while this is happening to you?

Sindu: He sits and watches in the same room, deriving total pleasure out of my pain. I wondered and wondered as to why he would derive this pleasure vicariously, until it dawned on me that he was impotent. What a disgustingly painful situation I walked into. (Shocked, soft sobs).

I let her sob and vent out.

Sindu: (Sighing) The same pattern again; it's my current life father who was my husband in that life.

Me: How does it make you feel?

Sindu: I'm done. I've forgiven him and I've forgiven myself. From my end, I've cut the loop. I'm neutral. Can we go forward? I want to learn my lesson of this brutal and sadistic life.

I appreciated that the wisdom of karmic connections had percolated deep into her and that brooding over it was no longer necessary for her. I chuckled quietly, again with appreciation, at her impatience as she was now very easily able to let go and move on 'fast' to the critical learnings. I also quietly reaffirmed that for regression therapy to be effective, the individual must embrace the knowledge and wisdom gained through exploration and keenly apply it to everyday practical life. This was a perfect example of such understanding practised sincerely and effectively. In line with her anticipation, I moved her on.

Me: How do you cope with this assault on an everyday basis?

Sindu: I use my mind to create a shield around me. I tell myself, 'Do whatever you want with me; nothing will affect me.'

This is exactly what she mentioned in the history session about the shield and I decided to focus on it and find out how it was connected with her body image.

Me: Focus on this shield. What is it like?

Sindu: This shield is like a bubble. My body, from my neck to knee, is encapsulated in this bubble. It is a thick fat layer about six feet away from my body. You rape, plunder, whip me, use nails on me ... anything, I will not feel it. This bubble allows me to disconnect my mind from my body. I refuse to feel anything. Even as my husband watched his guard approach me with lustful eyes, inflicting great pain on me, he sits smoking, smiling evilly, telling me, 'This will teach you. Beautiful girls must be taught a lesson.'

Me: How are you feeling?

Sindu: I am numb. I am fearless as I am insulated. I am separate from my body.

Me: Move forward to the next significant moment.

Sindu: My husband is ailing. I have one new fear in me. If my husband passes on, the savage guard will have total control over me.

Me: Why is the guard so torturous to you?

Sindu: Until my husband brought me home, his man guard thought that he would be the sole heir to all his wealth.

Me: Move forward to the next significant moment and get impressions.

Sindu: I'm thirty-four. My husband has died of a stroke. His will is being read. My stomach is churning with fear and disgust of this fear. And wonder of wonders, my husband has left everything to me. The first thing I do is to throw the savage out of my premises. Money brings me great physical security.

I have always been a person who derives great pleasure out of intellect. Born to an unwed mother and orphaned as a newborn, I've never been cuddled, crooned or kissed. I don't know the kind of affection and love that is associated with the body. Books have always been my refuge and the desire to think deeply and wisely coupled with simple living.

Me: And how are you moving forward after this escape?

Sindu: Now is my time. I do a lot of charity work and am feeling purposeful with these engagements.

Me: Do you continue to remain single?

Sindu: Yes. Many men flirt, show interest and even propose. I reject them. I am numb in my body and don't trust men anymore.

Me: Move forward.

Sindu: I am fifty-five years old. I keep myself busy. But, my eyes and soul feel empty. I am tired. I develop a fever and pass on, leaving all the wealth I inherited and built on further to many orphanages. I died alone, feeling no love, no companionship, numb to all the joys of life.

Me: Extending the moment of death, what are your affirmations as you die?

Sindu: My mind is totally twisted. I feel that I should not have been beautiful. It is better to be ugly; it helps to avoid attracting negative attention. There is a mantra in me ... hide the body, hide the beauty and you are safe. Do not attract negative attention. Never be happy with your body. Work only with the mind. My body should turn off other people. It is very important that whoever is with me, is genuinely for me and not just for my physical body.

I let her die, and ask about the reflection of the soul after looking at the whole life.

> Soul: The biggest problem was that I kept resigning to my fate when I should have taken some help and found a way out. But, I refused. In the beginning, when I used to contemplate on how to escape from the clutches of my venomous husband and his violent lustful man guard, I would immediately close my mind. My biggest worry was that if I escaped, my husband would not provide the orphanage with money; I feared that he would even find a way to take back the money he had given them. With time, I completely resigned to the life I was trapped in and even began to operate out of the conviction that I am not entitled to pleasure and happiness and that my beauty was a curse.

Me: How does this connect with your current life?

> Soul: My relationship with my body in my current life is also one of rebellion and torture. I live out of my body in this life too. Every time I have wanted to look good, maintain a fit, proportionate and vibrant body, the body fights back. I've been living my own curse of 'it is a punishment to look good' in this life.

Me: You had a reason to create it in that life, but do you need to keep it?

Sindu: No (very affirmative voice).

Me: What do you want to do with the shield?

Sindu: I just want to drop the shield that is surrounding me, and want to breathe free.

Me: What do you want to do with the oath, 'beauty is a curse'?

Sindu: (Breathing softly) It doesn't apply to me anymore.

She connected with me, a month later, happy to share some remarkable improvements. A few days after this session, in a quasi-awake state, in the wee hours of dawn, she felt a sheath floating away from her. She was certain that it was the physical manifestation of her release or catharsis. Within two weeks, most of her symptoms of pain improved. The true test of the release and the integration of the wisdom into her body was at the time of the lockdown enforced during the COVID-19 pandemic. She was able to do all the chores in the house and felt her body buzzing with the energy of a twenty-five-year-old. She said that she was falling in love with her body.

That is exactly the kind of cooperation I solicit from my clients on their healing journey. Be aware, apply the past knowledge to make the most of the present, and become responsible for your own lives: healing will automatically unfold.

III

ADDENDUM

Questions and Answers on Regression Therapy

When and how did regression therapy originate? Who is/are the founder/s of this modality of healing?
The origin of regression therapy as a modality of healing can be traced back to the Dream Incubation Schools of ancient Egypt and Greece. Then there were also the ancient Greek and Egyptian Mystery Schools, which provided access to the past lives of individuals. Regression therapy as a healing method drew a lot from the work and findings in the field of psychoanalysis by Sigmund Freud, the famous psychologist of the nineteenth century, and he inspires much of its current form.

Freud may be termed as the Grand Daddy of regression therapy. He was the first person to propagate to the world that the subconscious, if brought to the individual's consciousness and awareness, has the potential to heal. Before Freud, the psychologist largely depended on hypnosis to access the subconscious, but the art of hypnosis, then, was not as refined as it is today. When Freud realised that he could not take his clients effectively into a state of trance through hypnosis, he resorted to the art and science of Free Association[1] to tap into the subconscious minds of his clients. This technique of Free Association is what is largely used in regression therapy today.

Then we have Carl Jung, in the twentieth century, who started accessing past memories from the human subconscious with the help of active imagination. Edgar Cayce, too, was known for acting as a channel to access the past lives of other individuals. In a cruder way, in the 1950s, Stanislav Grof started using Lysergic Acid Diethylamide (LSD) to access memories of individuals associated with the womb, that is, the prenatal experiences or foetal memories. His work and experiments in the field of Transpersonal Psychology shook and shocked the scientific community of that era: *When there are neurons yet to be formed, that is, when the neurons are not yet myelinated, how can memories be retained or stored by the foetus?*

The next form of regression, also in 1950, came with Dianetics, a movement popularised by the science fiction writer L. Ron Hubbard and largely followed by the supporters of Scientology and the Nation of Islam. Under this movement, the process of accessing past memories was called auditing. The drawback of this technique as a therapy was that it focused more on diagnosing rather than treating. Its focus was on finding out what memory from the past was affecting the individual's current situation, and letting them live with the trauma of whatever they explored through their subconscious, without integrating or giving a proper closure to the memory in the present. In such cases, the issues would largely be left unresolved, reducing the therapeutic effect of Dianetics.

These drawbacks were largely cleared through intense work in the field by Morris Netherton, the author of *Past Lives Therapy*. Netherton refined the process and means of tapping into the subconscious of the human mind and gaining access to past memories for healing in the present.

In 1960, Denys Kelsey, a British psychologist, and his intuitively gifted wife, Joan Grant, published their findings of past life regression in their revolutionary book, *Many Lifetimes*. Denys, a scientist himself, approached the subject of regression in a very scientific and research-oriented way. He challenged the scientific community by bringing out the hypothesis that we cannot deny the existence of something abstract just because of an absence of concrete proof. He was referring to the belief of having access to memories associated with past lives, and not just those from the past of the current life or foetal memories.

The revolutionary work of the British couple mentioned above, paved the way for many other therapists from the field of psychology, psychiatry, psychoanalysis and metaphysics to come forward and conduct research and work in regression therapy and, at the same time, use it as a therapeutic technique to heal their clients. These include the likes of Helen Wambach, Michael Newton, Chet Snow, Roger Woolger, Thorwald Dethlefsen, and so on.

Last but not the least, one cannot but refrain from mentioning and acknowledging Dr Brian Weiss, whose work and writings truly brought this modality of healing to the vision and accessibility of a very large mass of world population.

The word 'intuition' has been used throughout the book. What does it mean?

In lay terms, intuition can be simply defined as the voice of the heart. It is the sixth sense, as sometimes people like to call it. From my own experience as a mainstream doctor and therapist, as well as a layperson, I am convinced that it is the heart that is the seat of intuition. Now let us look at it from an empirical perspective.

The HeartMath Institute has been researching the physiological mechanism of the heart and how it communicates with the brain and processes information; it analyses emotions and how they are perceived or sensed. Among these, their landmark research is about a pre-stimulus response, which is nothing but the science of intuition. In one such very interesting study, conducted by the institute, different images capable of stimulating emotions like fear, joy, grief and so on, were displayed one after the other in front of a sample group of the population. The heart-rhythm activity, or the heart-rate variability (ECG), and the brain responses (EEG) were recorded in each case. It was observed that people were able to sense the emotion before the image was displayed.

While both the heart and the brain received the pre-stimulus information about four to five seconds before being exposed to a future emotional image randomly selected by the computer, the heart actually received the information 1.5 seconds before the brain.[2]

There are several other areas of study related to the heart, involving memory and energy fields. In my work as a therapist, when I take people into a deep subconscious state, there are some who reveal memories that go back as far as the time they were in their mother's womb, as a newly formed foetus. Medically speaking, pregnancy is confirmed when the heart of the new life inside the mother's womb starts beating. The brain is not yet formed in any way; it is just a primitive bunch of neurons at that time. But the heart of the foetus is pumping. So, when a person recollects and shares an episode which occurred that early in their life, what part of the human system is responsible for that memory?

In his groundbreaking work, *The Heart's Code*, Dr. Paul Pearsall cites several anecdotes on this topic. He combines ancient wisdom, modern education, and scientific research to demonstrate that the human heart holds the secret to the link between body, mind and spirit. His study focuses on the heart's memory and energy field, showing that the heart is not just a pumping organ, but also retains subtle information and is in, itself, a source of infinite knowledge yet to be discovered and comprehended by the science of modern times.

Similarly, there are instances when people in a coma are known to capture or perceive what is happening around them, and some of these episodes are termed Near Death Experiences (NDE). Anita Moorjani is a living example of mind over matter. In 2006, after a four-year battle with cancer, she fell into a coma and was given hours to live. As her doctors gathered to revive her, she journeyed into a near-death experience (NDE) where she was given the choice to return to her physical form or to continue into this new realm. She chose the former, and when she regained consciousness, her cancer began to heal.

To the amazement of her doctors, she was free of countless tumours and cancer indicators within weeks.

When a person is in coma, the brain function is minimal. In this state, Anita saw her whole life and had a complete experience out of the body. This indicates that just because science has not discovered or deciphered it yet, it doesn't mean that NDEs do not exist.

What part of the human system actually perceives these seemingly out-of-body sensations, when the brain activity is clinically nil or negligent? What I find even more fascinating is that, like the birth of the foetus in the mother's womb, the death of the person is medically certified only when the heart stops beating or functioning. It is an indication that the heart is not only the seat of intuition, but essentially the source or centre of life itself. Dr. Raymond Moody's *Life After Life* is a wonderful scientific treatise for those who wish to explore this subject in more depth.

The heart's wisdom is an ancient science. Shamans or elders in all cultures were well-versed in using their intuition to predict changes in the season or the weather, foretelling birth and death, and identifying nature's resources for healing and vitality. Even today, there are indigenous tribes around the world who are well-versed in the art of tapping into and using the heart's secret potential, which may appear incomprehensible and inaccessible to the scientific community of these modern times. Surely a lot more research needs to be done on this unassuming little organ, for I am certain the heart is not merely a physical pump and that there is a lot more to what is visible or tangible. It may hold the key to life, death, and perhaps even beyond.

Does every human being have the power of intuition? How can we tap into our intuitive potential?
Yes, *every human being* has the potential of tapping into their heart's wisdom or, in other words, using their intuitive capacity.

How to develop intuition? Well, simply by using it more and more. By listening and allowing oneself to be guided by the heart's voice, instead of shrugging it off as hocus-pocus.

How to cultivate listening to the heart's voice? How to access the wisdom of the heart?

In almost all cultures around the world, a person is described by the quality of their heart: 'Oh, he is such a kind-hearted man,' 'She is so warm-hearted,' or 'They are hard-hearted people.' So, if you want to change the nature or behaviour of a person, where is the change really needed? The answer seems obvious: the heart. And that is why the Heartfulness Institute recommends meditation on the heart, with the aid of a unique and ancient technique known as Yogic Transmission. You will find more details on Yogic Transmission and its benefits at https://www.heartfulnessmagazine.com/transmission/.

During pilot research with TerraBlue XT, we studied the flow of Yogic Transmission with the help of a device that records physiological functions of the body, while the person is involved in different activities like sleeping, resting, relaxing, or meditating. Our findings showed that there is certainly a flow of energy between the trainer's heart and the one receiving the Transmission, despite the absence of any physical contact between the two people in the meditative state. During every such meditation, the TerraBlue device recorded a positive shift in heart-rate variability and galvanic skin response, indicating that the people meditating were in a deep state of calm and rest.

Time and again, practitioners have shared the profound changes in their own nature and in their surrounding environment as a result of practicing Heartfulness techniques over a sustained period of time. You may read some of these articles at https://heartfulness.org/in/humans-ofheartfulness/.

In my own experience, I have found that a regular and systematic practice of the Heartfulness techniques help in developing the ability to discriminate. Through meditation on the heart, again and again, we are able to distinguish and differentiate clearly between the voice of the heart and the chatter of the mind. So, for those looking to develop your intuitive capacity, I strongly recommend learning the techniques of Heartfulness by contacting your nearest Heartfulness centre or Heartfulness trainer.

Can anyone, for that matter, become a regression therapist?
There is more of the common population today than ever before, who is willing to not only be treated or healed with the aid of this therapy but is also keen to learn the technique of regression to heal others. I personally know people who essentially do not have a medical, psychological or scientific education or professional background, like a housewife or a school teacher, but who have a deep passion for helping and healing others. And they have been able to develop their intuitive abilities to an extent that they are able to use this tool to learn regression as a therapy. This passion to heal and help others is a precursor to learning the art and science of regression therapy, according to me, no matter what background you come from.

Having said that, as a mainstream doctor myself, I also realise that having medical knowledge is a blessing. It is an extra tool that helps to differentiate problems in a clear-cut fashion. It helps to identify the nature of the client's problem. More than anything, it helps me determine whether the person *really* needs to go through regression therapy to heal.

It is not uncommon that I have clients approaching me for something quite superficial, for which I strongly feel their ongoing treatment of allopathy is enough. For example, once a lady came to me with complaints of aches and pains in her lower back. She said she had already undergone two sessions of past life therapy with another therapist but was yet to see any positive change in her lower back condition. When I examined her, I found that she had sacroiliac tenderness: there was a big knot in the muscles of her lower back. So, I probed deeper.

Me: How do you usually sit on the chair?

Client: I sit in a slouched position.

Me: Do you exercise?

Client: No.

Me: For how long do you watch television?

Client: On a daily basis, I watch TV at least for three hours.

Me: What job do you do?

Client: I am a software professional.

I told the lady that her problem lay in the *here and now*, and not in any past life. It was clear to me that she was not in need of any regression to cure her of her lower back pain. Instead of wasting her time in therapies, I suggested she started doing Yoga and indulge in other physical exercises to heal her back. She was wise to heed my advice. After four weeks, she called me and said that the pain in her lower back had completely vanished.

I strongly recommend having a medical background or acquiring medical knowledge, in order to be able to really do justice to your role as a regression therapist. Or at least get a professional opinion before starting therapy.

Is there any affiliated institute or professional course that can train you to become a professional regression therapist?
Yes, there are quite a number of training schools today that teach hypnotherapy, regression and past-life therapy.

Can anyone under the sky, or simply out of curiosity, go in for regression therapy?
This is like asking: Does every human being need to see a doctor?

The answer is: Of course not.

You visit a doctor only when you are facing some physical ailment or disorder. You see a psychologist or a psychiatrist when you are down with some kind of a mental or emotional problem. Similarly, I seriously do not recommend regression just for the sake of it or out of plain curiosity or for the sake of fun. That would be like the case of using a crane to pick a needle.

Regression is a life-changing process, and one needs to have a serious, rather a sacred approach to the therapy. Also, why would you be willing to waste your time and money to go to a therapist, unless you feel you are going to benefit out of it in some way?

The best time to try this modality of healing is when your physical or mental condition keeps persisting or relapsing in spite of trying out various treatments and medications. Most of my clients come with a history of medical diagnosis and treatments, which they may have followed for a period of time, before opting for regression therapy.

I strongly recommend regression therapy only after you have consulted a mainstream doctor, or your family physician, for your physical symptoms. If, after persistent consultation and treatment, you are unable to trace the cause of the disease or if the doctor terms the symptoms as idiopathic, then the root of the disorder may most likely lie in your mind or emotions. In that case, yes, you may consider regression therapy.

The only exception to the above is when the individual is seeking answers to repetitive patterns in their life with respect to their spiritual quest. I have had clients approaching me when they feel kind of 'stuck' in their spiritual journey owing to certain relationships, addictions, feeling of a void or incompleteness, deep personal grief or some kind of a trauma, and are seeking answers that may prove as an opening in their inner journey. Regression can be used effectively to address such issues too.

How can people who don't believe in past lives or reincarnation benefit from regression therapy?
I know it can be difficult to believe in this modality of healing, given our scientific or proof-oriented bent of mind, and especially if we're following a faith that doesn't advocate reincarnation or the existence of an eternal soul. It took me time, too, to develop conviction in this process; it did not happen overnight, as I am a firm believer of evidence-based medicine.

I have clients from different religious backgrounds who approach me with some amount of scepticism. When they express their disbelief or doubt in the therapy, I suggest they try giving it a shot with an open mind. There are no side-effects to regression when approached and facilitated in the right way and through the right person. The purpose of any therapy, ultimately, is healing, and the proof of the pudding lies in its eating. So why not give it a try, especially since you have tried all other conventional ways of curing without much result? You may start trusting the modality once you see the result of the therapy. And even if apparently positive results do not succeed in gaining your trust in the therapy, you still are free to term the healing as mental catharsis and simply acknowledge the potential of the mind.

In a nutshell, if the therapy works, you will be the happiest person on earth; if not, you have nothing to lose.

Most of my clients who approached regression with this attitude, irrespective of their beliefs or religion, have seen positive results after going through the sessions. While approximately 80 per cent of such sceptics actually regressed into past lives, the rest of them healed by dealing with the ghosts of their youth or childhood. Regression is not about past lives alone, and the therapy includes digging into the subconscious for emotions that may have been buried deep in your childhood or when you were younger. In fact, in my work, I have largely witnessed that fresh wounds hurt more than the older ones and hence dealing with the emotional charges or impression of the present life helps significantly. Regression basically means moving back in time, and that could even be a time that has passed in your present life.

Actually, when Denys Kelsey started using regression therapy, he was only looking for and expecting the surfacing of buried childhood memories. But when, in some of the sessions, clients went into memories that had no coherence with either their present life or with the foetal period, Kelsey was baffled. It did not make any sense to him and that is when he hit upon the hunch that these particular memories may perhaps have belonged to an altogether different lifetime than the present one. That is when he joined hands (and married at a later point in time) with Joan Grant, who was highly intuitive and seemed to carry memories of her past lives. The couple approached the theory and idea of reincarnation from various angles and did many studies and experiments together, finally coming up with a solid research-oriented backing to the science of regression. Their experiments and findings are part of their revolutionary book, *Many Lifetimes*, which was first published in 1967.

In another interesting instance, Ian Stevenson encountered and interviewed children who could recall their immediate past lives, as part of his work and research. After his session with each child, he would go in search of the place—village, town or city—find it, and speak to the locals of that place to find out if a person by the name that the child had described ever lived there. To his amazement, he got positive answers, which proved that the children whom he had interacted with, indeed, had had a lifetime in the past in that place.

Is it okay to continue with regular medicines and other treatments while you are going through regression therapy?
Yes, it is absolutely fine to do so. There is no harm in continuing your ongoing treatment, whether homoeopathy, Ayurveda,

allopathy, or any other modality of healing, along with regression therapy.

If clients are already on medication, I do not recommend them to discontinue the dosage abruptly or immediately. I wait and watch for the results or progress in the client's condition after every session. The follow-up happens daily, weekly, monthly or yearly, as needed. As I see their condition improving, I slowly taper down the dosage of the oral medicines and if needed, even advise them to stop completely. In some other cases, it may take longer to wean the patient away from their oral medication, as they may take a while to imbibe the lessons that emerge through regression into their present life, and thereby benefit out of the therapy.

Here, again, my medical background proves really handy.

How many sessions does a person need of regression therapy?
This is like walking into the doctor's clinic and asking him or her: How long will it take for the fever to go away? The doctor may give you a probable time frame depending on the diagnosis. And in most cases, he or she may ask you to come for a follow-up meeting after a few days to decide whether you are cured or you need further treatment.

Similarly, the number of sessions that a client needs depends on how deep-rooted the problem is. For example, you may pull out a small sapling out of the soil with just two fingers of your hand. But can you do the same to uproot a giant tree, whose roots have gone deep into the soil?

Over a period of time, and after dealing with over a thousand clients, I have understood that I can never determine at the onset, the number of sessions that a particular person may need for healing to result in a holistic way. Though fewer in number, there are some cases where the client heals completely just after one session of regression. But in most of the cases, the manifesting physical condition is just the tip of the iceberg. It is only when I review the client during a follow-up session that the next layer of the problem surfaces, like peeling an onion, layer after layer.

That's why follow-up sessions are such an important and integral part of regression therapy. At the very onset, you can never determine how many sessions a client may need to go through to heal completely.

What is trance? How can one take clients into a state of trance?
Etymologically, the word 'trance' means to 'go across'. A common meaning of the word is 'a semi-conscious state, in which the person seems to be asleep but is aware of what is being spoken around and said to them'. Even in our day-to-day life, we may go into this kind of a dazed state, induced by some kind of an external (or internal) stimulus, without the awareness of being in a trance. For example, have you seen children watching their favourite cartoon programme on television? Eyes glued to the TV set, motionless body, and totally oblivious to any other noise around; then, they don't even hear the shouting and yelling of their parents!

According to research, this state of being, where you are neither fully conscious nor fully unconscious, is most conducive to tap into the subconscious. Hence, it becomes necessary for therapists to be able to take their clients into a trance in order to access past memories. Of course, there are many ways and means by which you can induce a person into the state of trance. While hypnosis is a common tool used by many therapists for this purpose, I personally do not use the technique often.

Half of my work with the client happens during the history-taking session, where I probe and dig deep to gain clarity about what is *really* bothering the person. I try to identify the core issue, the core emotion, the core feeling associated with the manifesting issue, by asking them relevant questions. While conversing in this manner, I am very attentive to the body language of the person.

Almost all the time, when the core emotion feeding the manifesting issue emerges, I observe a physical reaction in the person's body. The physical reaction could be anything, from facial expressions to shrugging the shoulders or squirming of the body, and it suggests something significant. As I help them to connect with their physical body, most of the time there is a specific physical reaction that acts as a bridge to take them into a state of trance. This 'bridge' may take a non-physical form too, that is, it may not necessarily involve the physical body or emotions, but may just be a postulate: *I can never trust anyone.* At times, the client may even begin to cry or their voice becomes shaky, and then I know I have hit upon something: the person has either started accessing the memory or is living it again in his or her mind.

I use such 'bridges'—by grounding my clients into their physical selves by identifying the physical reactions, the feeding emotions and associated feeling—to take them into a state of trance. Once this is done, I generally ask them to close their eyes, feel their body, and their breath, and usually they slip into a trance with just a few suggestions. I create a safe imaginative space, where the client feels comfortable, and intensify the feeling or the emotion associated with the manifesting issue as a bridge. They are made to repeat this a few times, and then I count backwards to help them cross over from *this* time to *that* time, the time when their present manifesting issue first began. *What is the first impression surfacing?*

This technique of taking the client into a state of trance, using their very problem as the tool and without spending much time in relaxing them initially (which is what hypnosis aims at, and that is why many therapists resort to the technique as a tool to 'cross over' in regression), is easier but comes with a lot of practice.

How do you know that you are *actually* 'seeing' your past, or going through the experience of reliving your past, and that it is not just a play of your mind or imagination?
When I started practising the therapy, I had the same doubt: Was the client really going through a past experience, or was it just the mind working at its creative best?

One way to answer this question is by observing the client's body language when he or she is in a state of trance. The physical body usually does not lie; it carries and manifests the trauma of any past memory. Whenever the client is able to access a past memory through regression, they also relive the strongest emotion associated with that memory. And in almost all cases, the emotion causes some change in the person's body language, even when they are in a subconscious state during the session. These changes in the body of the client can surface and be witnessed in the form of pain, heaviness, tightness or numbness in some part of the body. At times, you can really *see* or feel the client's heartbeat going faster; or sometimes, the client starts scratching some part of the body; or just makes some weird facial expressions.

In reality, during regression, your whole body feels and senses *exactly* the same experience as the time when it was undergoing that particular experience, which you are trying to access from your subconscious. For example, if you are reliving the memory of someone stabbing you at a particular spot on your body, you may experience a piercing pain exactly at the same spot during your regression session.

Once, a lady from a Catholic background approached me just because her close friend had recommended and raved about the benefits of regression therapy. She was suffering from chronic fatigue syndrome, fibromyalgia and severe depression. She told me openly that she did not believe in past lives and that she had come to see me as a last resort, after trying all other treatments and on the strong recommendation of her friend. She said, 'I don't believe in all this, but I will do what you ask me to do. If you want me to close my eyes, I shall close my eyes.'

To the lady's utter bewilderment, and to mine too, within a very few minutes she had floated into a state of trance and had crossed over to a past lifetime. Even from that subconscious state, she kept telling me that she was unable to believe what she was 'seeing', and kept wondering aloud if it was all real or imagination. Suddenly this woman, who was from the beginning quite animated in her expressions, froze on the recliner. She was not able to move her hands and legs, and said that she felt very, very tired all of a sudden. The session lasted for four hours. My sceptical client had successfully regressed into a lifetime where she had been paralysed, and thus her motionless body on my recliner at the time of regression. Needless to say, she made a complete recovery within two months and still cannot get over being amazed about it.

Can regression therapy effectively cure people ailing from mental or psychological disorders? Is there any specific group of people for whom you may not recommend regression as a modality of healing?
Regression therapy is a process where you use your mind to heal yourself. So, the primary criterion for this therapy to work is that you should be *able and willing* to use your mind in a sane and discriminative way. In the light of this underlying fact, regression cannot be used to treat individuals suffering from psychosis, as they have primarily lost touch with reality. Practically speaking, they won't be able to go through the process involved in the therapy and so the question of healing through regression doesn't arise.

In the case of clients who are down with acute depression, I make my judgements whether they would really benefit out of regression or not only after spending enough time interacting with them to understand how fit they are in their minds to actually cooperate in bringing about their own healing.

Similarly, I would not recommend this therapy for people under the influence of drugs. Most of the time they are not willing to be healed, and they mostly approach a therapist or a rehabilitation centre on the insistence of their family, friends and well-wishers. They generally do not wish to come out of their addiction and hence do not actively seek to be helped.

Then there are the control freaks, for whom it becomes tough to even get to the state of trance, or a subconscious state, as they do not want to expose themselves and hence block the therapist from accessing their minds and memories. In that case, too, regression therapy becomes difficult. In fact, it would be wiser to get to the root of their controlling nature or behaviour and help them in letting go of that in the first place. It is a lot like opening the lock first before gaining access.

The last category consists of people who do not want to take responsibility for their actions and cooperate with the therapist in healing. They feel they are the victims all the time and, hence, keep indulging in self-pity. Regression therapy does not prove useful or beneficial to such people.

Is regression therapy safe for children? Can they be adversely affected by what they 'see' during the sessions?
Yes, it is very safe for children to undergo regression therapy.

As parents it is natural to feel concerned whether your child will be able to relive the traumatic experience that may most likely surface during regression. In my career, the youngest individual whom I did regression on directly, and not through surrogacy, was four years old. And she healed through the therapy.

In my work with children, I have observed a common pattern: if the memory associated with the manifesting physical condition is traumatic to the extent that the child is not able to handle it, they automatically 'refuse' to open up during the session. *I don't see anything. I cannot see anything.* That is because the mind is not yet ready to reveal and is smart enough to block the memory! And when they *are* ready to handle the situation, their minds naturally open up, giving them access to the memory.

I remember an eight-year-old boy with severe asthma, who didn't 'see' anything during the first session. My therapy couldn't really do anything about his condition at that time. But when he was eleven year old, he came back, and this time he just seemed ready to go through the process. I was able to regress him successfully and subsequently, he was relieved of asthma.

It's beautiful to witness how children are able to protect themselves in this manner. That's also the beauty of the healing power of the mind.

People at large may be scared that they may never be able to get over a past memory awakened through regression. Doctors may also be concerned about situations where the patient is not able to get over a very traumatic memory that is likely to surface during regression, and in the process, they may continue to undergo the trauma of the past. What solution, or precaution, can be taken in these types of cases?

In general, most of my clients seeking regression as therapy do so only after they have exhausted many other options of treatment. I have observed that by the time they approach me for regression, they are somehow prepared and willing to face whatever it takes to heal. And this in itself brings an attitude of courage. The ones who are scared or hesitant are mostly those who haven't come out of their own willingness, but are coerced into trying a session by a family member or persuaded by a doctor, and most don't return after the history session. Even if they do, they refuse to go into a state of trance. If somehow, they cooperate and *do* manage to go through a session, then acceptance of the past and learning and taking responsibility to bring the learning into action, which is the *most vital* step expected on the part of the client for complete healing to occur, remains lacking.

Freud believed that when we bring the unknown to the known mind, it helps in the healing of people (or healing of the trauma). There is a science as to how such healing happens in regression therapy. Let me explain the process in a little detail below:

A memory is awakened and relived with the willingness of the person, and an understanding is arrived upon with the help of a skilled therapist. The understanding is integrated into the conscious mind, paving the way for new wisdom, which allows people to tame their ego, pin the responsibility for their challenge correctly (either on themselves, or on the other person in the case of abusive and toxic relationships) and accept the situation from a wiser state of being.

When people are able to see themselves in alternative roles of being a victim as well as a person causing hurt to somebody else across lives (the victimiser), the opposites neutralise and the equation usually balances out. The sessions mostly end with the therapist guiding the client to release all emotions that are detrimental, such as anger, hate, fear, injustice and so on, consciously, willingly, and with full awareness. When this sequence of awakening, understanding, integration and release—a dance between the condition of the client and the intuition and skill of the therapist—is executed correctly, there is no fear or trauma in the person going forward. In fact, there is a new understanding and wisdom, and this paves the way for the beginning of healing.

I emphasise on *beginning*, as there is one more step for the process to be complete—and that is through spontaneous healing. For a few days after the session, depending on what has been relived, the person may go through certain raw emotions and perhaps even extreme physical fatigue and fever. These are signs of an effective session, as the right chord has been struck and the body is in the phase of releasing all toxic residues to heal. Gradually, the acquired wisdom kicks in, newer perspectives towards the very same life unfold, memories of the past fade, and only the lessons to be learnt and the shifts to be made prevail, allowing the person to move forward. The entire process could take weeks or months, depending on the individual's capacity to heal.

The fading of the memory of the past relived during regression, which is a big part of the question, can be understood with the help of a metaphor. Think of a huge balloon occupying a whole room. Now imagine puncturing the balloon and releasing the air. When all the air is released, what happens to the balloon? How does it appear now? Can you view it in the same way as it was earlier, big and occupying the whole room? The answer obviously is no. In place of the big, bloated balloon, you may now see a small, shrivelled sliver of a balloon lying in a corner of the room. It is there, but not in your direct visibility, and even if you are able to spot it, you see it just as a shrivelled piece.

This is exactly what happens to the memory: the release and integration and healing let the trauma out of the memory, shrivelling it to a discarded faint memory, which has no effect on the person. All of this happens naturally, with a deeper willingness and the application of the will of the individual.

Both the therapist and the person are equally responsible for healing to be effective. Healing may prove incomplete if the therapist does not execute even one step in this sequence properly and completely. On the other hand, if a person after experiencing the understanding shows resistance to this new learning, and does not accept and chooses to remain in blame, self-pity or victim mode, healing is incomplete.

As a therapist, I rely very much on my understanding of the client while talking to him or her, on common sense, and on my intuition and experiences of the client who I agree to heal through regression. If I feel that the person may not cooperate, I do not take responsibility for their actions. If I find their ego too rigid or I find them indulging in too much of self-pity, I generally avoid suggesting and treating them through regression therapy.

IV

INSIGHTS

The Science of Mind Over Matter

A shift in the modality or process, in any existing system, is very much in response to changing times. What is interesting to observe and note is whether these radical changes follow a linear or circular pattern in time. Consider the medical scenario five decades ago. Specialists and super specialists in the field were almost unheard of, and we were likely to come across 'family doctors' who were well-versed in playing the role of agony aunts more than anything else. A patient listening to the patient's woes was very much a part of the treatment meted out, the medicine probably acting just as a placebo. So, did people not heal and recover then?

In the last few decades, there has been a paradigm shift in the way we approach the idea of healing. Justifiably replaced with the word 'treatment', I regret to state that healing today is not as holistic as it used to be and should be. As a physician, the more you specialise in one aspect of a disease, the more is your worth and credibility among both the fraternity as well as the community of patients. Instead of viewing the disease as a whole, we are specialists at dissecting it into several parts, each calling for a different channel of treatment.

Take the case of a person suffering from Systemic Lupus Erythematosus. In today's age, she would be ideally guided to consult a nephrologist for the functioning of her kidney; a rheumatologist to examine her joints; a gastroenterologist to eliminate the possibility of a disorder with her stomach; a neurologist for psychosis; a haematologist for treating low blood count; and last but not the least, a general physician to advise her on whatever may be left out, if at all anything. Being caught in this web of specialisation myself, I would without any qualms assert that psychologists do a better job in trying to find out what has actually been going wrong with their client's life, or lifestyle, for the manifestation of the physical disorder. They give the patients a patient hearing, and that helps at least to some extent depending on various factors.

Added to these internal woes of medical and health services, mass conditioning today plays a very big role in magnifying the fear associated with any disease and its impact on peoples' minds. During my interaction with clients and patients, I have observed that the ones who respond speedily and positively to any kind of treatment, leave alone regression, are the ones who have the toughest minds. *They have the will to heal, so they heal.*

The dire need for doctors and healthcare providers today, as well as for the future, as I see it, is to view the patient and their disease as one whole. And alternative therapies, such as regression, are of great help to bring about this kind of integration in the approach. We need to open up to the idea of using these indigenous sciences as an adjuvant or an auxiliary to work synergistically with allopathy in healing patients, especially in the case of chronic diseases. For example, conditions such as rheumatoid arthritis can be very effectively dealt with through this combined approach. Allopathic medicines can be administered to the patient to momentarily relieve the terrible pain in their joints, and at the same time we can address the root cause of the problem through regression so that permanent healing and recovery is successfully facilitated. Come to think of it, alternative therapies are not unheard of in allopathy, especially now with more and more medical centres and hospitals opening their doors to such ideas and concepts as part of their units.

A very valid question at this juncture would be: Is regression the only science that can be integrated in this manner with conventional treatment for holistic healing? I really cannot answer that; however, what I can empirically state is that any practice or modality which has the potential of using and stimulating the mind to heal is worthy of consideration. I'd like to refer to them as 'the science of mind over matter'.

When a person goes through regression, and understands the cause of their present suffering, they are faced with the real task of participating in the healing process by forgiving or making peace with their past and learning from it. Contrary to what some of us may perceive it as, regression is not mumbo-jumbo where transformation occurs at the wave of a wand, but it is a very potent science in which we use the very instrument which sets us apart from all other species of life: the mind. It requires the patient or the client to consciously work with their minds to heal themselves, with the assistance of the therapist as a facilitator.

For the same reason, many go through regression but do not apply the wisdom gained out of it in their present lives, and they fall short of holistic healing or total recovery. In some cases, the physical symptoms manifest again, and the cause for these is contained in the science that backs this modality of healing.

When we go through regression, we gain an understanding in our mind of the cause of our troubles in our current state and time, so that we are aware and alert when the same pattern of the past presents itself again in the present. We now not only have an understanding but every part of our body has a feel of the past memory and experience. We can then heal ourselves by creating new neural pathways in our mind, of understanding, approaching and dealing with our past in the present and the present through our past.

Forming new neural pathways is like opening a new chapter or page in life, which gives us the opportunity to refill ourselves with hope, faith and enthusiasm that add a fresh lease of life to our existence. One of my clients revealed, 'I find that when I forget to follow the new neural pathway and lapse into my old ways of thinking, even after I have gone through regression and made peace with my past, the body symptoms come back. I have to remind myself that I need to use this new pathway in my mind and help it integrate into my body.'

My greatest challenge so far has been to overcome the solid barrier of the notion that allopathy is the supreme science in medicine. I don't deny that it is the best for acute conditions and emergencies; it very much is. But when it comes to chronic conditions, we need to understand that an alternative therapy like regression definitely helps explore the mind to find out the root cause of the disease or disorder. *We need to look beyond what is visible or apparent.* Look beyond what is manifested, not just go by symptoms, and try to locate the fire that is emitting the smoke. What is the use of clearing the smoke when its source has been left unattended, un-extinguished? And that is also the biggest takeaway from my time spent in the field of medicine: delve into the root cause of the disease instead of superficially treating it just on the basis of the symptoms or diagnosis.

I urge you all to consider regression therapy as a new science or modality that helps us heal with no side-effects. The most important quality for all those who wish to heal—and for the healers themselves—is to have an open mind, for, then comes the opportunities to learn and unlearn. Each day carries the potential to grant us new experiences and lessons. Regression is an alchemical science, helping us to evolve from surviving to living and to loving. Its success depends on how much we are willing to let go.

Acknowledgements

I would like to thank all my clients who have helped me refine myself as a therapist and as a human being, with all the healing they went through and the emerging wisdom.

I also would like to thank those clients who did not benefit from the therapy, for their criticism helped me refine myself and my approach.

I am deeply grateful to all my spiritual guides and teachers, especially Chariji, who groomed me. And to my loving family who are a constant invaluable support.

Last but not least, I would like to thank two wonderful friends (who wish to remain anonymous) who helped me complete this book.

www.ingramcontent.com/pod-product-compliance
Lightning Source LLC
LaVergne TN
LVHW041939070526
838199LV00051BA/2842